Obstetric Anesthesia

Editor

ROBERT GAISER

ANESTHESIOLOGY CLINICS

www.anesthesiology.theclinics.com

Consulting Editor
LEE A. FLEISHER

September 2013 • Volume 31 • Number 3

ELSEVIER

1600 John F. Kennedy Boulevard • Suite 1800 • Philadelphia, Pennsylvania, 19103-2899

http://www.theclinics.com

ANESTHESIOLOGY CLINICS Volume 31, Number 3
September 2013 ISSN 1932-2275, ISBN-13: 978-0-323-18842-5

Editor: Jennifer Flynn-Briggs

Anesthesiology Clinics (ISSN 1932-2275) is published quarterly by Elsevier Inc., 360 Park Avenue South, New York, NY 10010-1710. Months of issue are March, June, September, and December. Periodicals postage paid at New York, NY and at additional mailing offices. Subscription prices are $154.00 per year (US student/resident), $313.00 per year (US individuals), $383.00 per year (Canadian individuals), $516.00 per year (US institutions), $639.00 per year (Canadian institutions), $216.00 per year (Canadian and foreign student/resident), $434.00 per year (foreign individuals), and $639.00 per year (foreign institutions). To receive student and resident rate, orders must be accompanied by name of affiliated institution, date of term, and the *signature* of program/residency coordinator on institutions letterhead. Orders will be billed at individual rate until proof of status is received. Foreign air speed delivery is included in all *Clinics'* subscription prices. All prices are subject to change without notice. POSTMASTER: Send address changes to *Anesthesiology Clinics,* Elsevier Health Sciences Division, Subscription Customer Service, 3251 Riverport Lane, Maryland Heights, MO 63043. Customer Service (orders, claims, online, change of address): Elsevier Health Sciences Division, Subscription Customer Service, 3251 Riverport Lane, Maryland Heights, MO 63043. Tel:1-800-654-2452 (U.S. and Canada); 314-447-8871 (outside U.S. and Canada). Fax: 314-447-8029. E-mail: journalscustomerservice-usa@elsevier.com (for print support); journalsonlinesupport-usa@elsevier.com (for online support).

Reprints. For copies of 100 or more of articles in this publication, please contact the Commercial Reprints Department, Elsevier Inc., 360 Park Avenue South, New York, NY 10010-1710. Tel.: 212-633-3874; Fax: 212-633-3820; E-mail: reprints@elsevier.com.

Anesthesiology Clinics, is also published in Spanish by McGraw-Hill Inter-americana Editores S. A., P.O. Box 5-237, 06500 Mexico D. F., Mexico.

Anesthesiology Clinics, is covered in *MEDLINE/PubMed (Index Medicus), Current Contents/Clinical Medicine, Excerpta Medica, ISI/BIOMED,* and *Chemical Abstracts.*

Printed and bound by CPI Group (UK) Ltd, Croydon, CR0 4YY

Transferred to digital print 2013

Contributors

CONSULTING EDITOR

LEE A. FLEISHER, MD, FACC, FAHA
Robert D. Dripps Professor and Chair of Anesthesiology and Critical Care, Professor of Medicine, Perelman School of Medicine, University of Pennsylvania School of Medicine, Philadelphia, Pennsylvania

EDITOR

ROBERT GAISER, MD, MSEd
Professor, Department of Anesthesiology and Critical Care, University of Pennsylvania, Philadelphia, Pennsylvania

AUTHORS

HERSIMREN BASI, MD
Resident, Department of Anesthesiology, Western Pennsylvania Hospital, West Penn Allegheny Health System, Pittsburgh, Pennsylvania

CURTIS L. BAYSINGER, MD
Associate Professor, Director of Obstetric Anesthesia, Division of Obstetric Anesthesia, Department of Anesthesiology, Vanderbilt University Medical Center, Nashville, Tennessee

TAMMY EULIANO, MD
Associate Professor of Anesthesiology and Obstetrics and Gynecology, University of Florida College of Medicine, Gainesville, Florida

HELENE FINEGOLD, MD
Associate Professor of Anesthesiology, Department of Anesthesiology, Western Pennsylvania Hospital, West Penn Allegheny Health System, Pittsburgh, Pennsylvania

REGINA Y. FRAGNETO, MD
Professor of Anesthesiology and Director, Obstetric Anesthesia; Department of Anesthesiology, University of Kentucky College of Medicine, Lexington, Kentucky

ROBERT GAISER, MD, MSEd
Professor, Department of Anesthesiology and Critical Care, University of Pennsylvania, Philadelphia, Pennsylvania

WENDY A. HAFT, MD
Resident in Anesthesiology, Department of Anesthesiology, UPMC, Pittsburgh, Pennsylvania

JOHN M. KISSKO III, MD
Instructor, Department of Anesthesiology and Critical Care, University of Pennsylvania, Philadelphia, Pennsylvania

M. FAITH LUKENS, MD
Assistant Professor of Anesthesiology, Department of Anesthesiology, University of Kentucky College of Medicine, Lexington, Kentucky

ELAINE PAGES-ARROYO, MD
Department of Anesthesia, Brigham and Women's Hospital, Boston, Massachusetts

MAY C.M. PIAN-SMITH, MD, MS
Assistant Professor of Anesthesia, Harvard Medical School; Department of Anesthesia, Critical Care and Pain Medicine, Massachusetts General Hospital, Boston, Massachusetts

ABHA A. SHAH, MD
Assistant Professor, Department of Anesthesiology, University of Kansas Medical Center, Kansas City, Kansas

GRACE H. SHIH, MD
Associate Professor, Director of Obstetric Anesthesia, Department of Anesthesiology, University of Kansas Medical Center, Kansas City, Kansas

SARAH A. STARR, MD
Assistant Professor, Division of Obstetric Anesthesia, Department of Anesthesiology, Vanderbilt University Medical Center, Nashville, Tennessee

CHRISTOPHER A. TROIANOS, MD
Chairman and Professor of Anesthesiology, Department of Anesthesiology, Western Pennsylvania Hospital, West Penn Allegheny Health System, Pittsburgh, Pennsylvania

MANUEL C. VALLEJO, MD, DMD
Professor of Anesthesiology and Director of Obstetric Anesthesia, Department of Anesthesiology, Magee-Womens Hospital of UPMC, Pittsburgh, Pennsylvania

JASON D. WALLS, MD
Resident, Department of Anesthesiology and Critical Care, Hospital of the University of Pennsylvania, Philadelphia, Pennsylvania

Contents

Chronic pain may develop after surgery or trauma. It is defined as pain that persists for 2 months after the initial injury. Although the exact mechanism for the development of chronic pain is not understood, several risk factors have been identified, including female sex, older age, and certain surgical procedures. Chronic pain after cesarean or vaginal delivery has a reported incidence of 10% to 15%. Given the large number of cesarean sections performed, this incidence is concerning. However, a recent study by academic anesthesiologists established the incidence to be much lower than expected.

Magnesium is an intracellular cation that functions as a cofactor in many biological processes, including calcium channel gating, release of neurotransmitters, modulation of vasomotor tone, and regulation of energy reactions. The role of magnesium in such processes makes it clinically applicable in many situations, especially obstetric practice. However, these same functions also result in the side effects and drug interactions associated with magnesium use, and, thus, necessitate careful administration. Peripartum use of magnesium sulfate has been well studied for tocolysis, preeclampsia and the prevention of progression to eclampsia, antiepileptic treatment in eclampsia, and neuroprotection of fetuses during preterm labor.

New airway techniques are especially relevant to the obstetric patient requiring anesthesia. Although regional anesthesia is the preferred mode of analgesia for vaginal delivery and of anesthesia for cesarean section, there are scenarios where tracheal intubation is required. Sometimes these cases are anticipated but more often are emergent, and tracheal intubation may be unexpectedly difficult. An unanticipated emergent difficult airway in the labor suite is perhaps the highest stress situation for the anesthesiologist. Anesthesiologists must be proficient in a wide variety of advanced airway techniques with a thorough understanding of emergent airway algorithms, and familiarization with the newest airway devices.

Amniotic fluid embolism (AFE) is a rare and lethal clinical syndrome. The classic triad of AFE is cardiovascular collapse, respiratory distress, and disseminated intravascular coagulopathy. The understanding of its pathophysiology has changed since it was first described more than 85 years ago, and is now better described as an anaphylactoid reaction of pregnancy. Despite continued investigation into new methods of diagnosis, such as transesophageal echocardiography and insulin-like growth factor binding protein 1, and treatment modalities including intralipid and recombinant factor VIIa, AFE remains one of the major causes of maternal morbidity and mortality in the United States.

The use of inhaled nitrous oxide for labor analgesia is uncommon but increasing in the United States. It is widely used in several European countries and in Australia and New Zealand. The history of its use for the relief of pain during labor and its efficacy and side effects compared with other methods of labor analgesia are presented. Special equipment is necessary for its safe administration.

ANESTHESIOLOGY CLINICS

RELATED INTEREST

Obstetrics and Gynecology Clinics, September 2012 (Volume 39, Issue 3)
Collaborative Practice in Obstetrics and Gynecology
Richard Waldman, MD, FACOG and
Holly Powell Kennedy, PhD, CNM, FACNM, FAAN, *Editors*

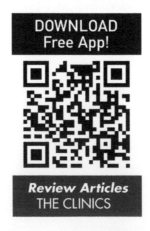

NOW AVAILABLE FOR YOUR iPhone and iPad

Preface

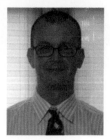

Robert Gaiser, MD, MSEd
Editor

Obstetric anesthesia continues to evolve. Previous problems of dense epidural blockade with possible increased risk of operative delivery have been solved. As old problems are solved, new ones are generated. It is important to examine these new problems because by discussing and exploring these concerns, solutions may be formulated. This issue presents these problems in obstetric anesthesia. Chronic pain in obstetrics, the effect of anesthesia and analgesia on the fetus's ability to learn, epidural analgesia as a source of maternal fever, and communication among providers have recently been identified as key issues in obstetric anesthesia. All of these topics were not even considered five years ago. Other problems, such as the use of magnesium, amniotic fluid embolism, and neurologic complications, continue to evolve with different solutions or different uses. Finally, issues that were thought to be settled have resurfaced as new investigation into its use has settled previous concerns, such as the use of nitrous oxide for the management of analgesia during labor. It is these problems and approaches to problems that make obstetric anesthesia such a fascinating specialty. It is both to these investigators that examine these concerns in obstetric anesthesia and to the reader who wants to learn more about obstetric anesthesia that this issue is dedicated.

ACKNOWLEDGMENT

I would like to acknowledge the continued support of my chairman, Dr Lee Fleisher, who motivates every member of the department and who is a true role model.

Robert Gaiser, MD, MSEd
Department of Anesthesiology and Critical Care
University of Pennsylvania
3400 Spruce Street
Philadelphia, PA 19104, USA

E-mail address:
Robert.gaiser@uphs.upenn.edu

Chronic Pain in the Obstetric Patient

Jason D. Walls, MD*, Robert Gaiser, MD, MSEd

KEYWORDS

- Chronic pain • Cesarean delivery • Vaginal delivery • Multimodal analgesia

KEY POINTS

- Chronic pain after surgery is pain that persists 2 months after the surgical incision.
- The progression from acute to chronic pain in certain individuals is unclear, but involves central nervous system centralization.
- Although several risk factors have been identified, the one consistently identified in studies is poorly managed acute postoperative pain.
- Given the risk factors, one would expect to have a high incidence of chronic pain after cesarean or vaginal delivery.
- The incidence of chronic pain after cesarean or vaginal delivery is much lower than expected.

INTRODUCTION

Chronic pain is a condition that may occur after any damage to a nerve. This condition is also known as *surgically induced neuropathic pain*, and consists of pain that persists beyond 2 months after the injury.[1] Why certain individuals develop chronic pain after acute pain from an injury is unclear. Certain injuries are more prone to the development of the syndrome than others. Chronic pain or surgically induced neuropathic pain occurs in 60% of patients after limb amputation,[2] 30% of patients after mastectomy,[3] 20% of patients after thoracotomy,[4] and in 20% of patients after hernia repair.[5] Given these occurrences, one may expect chronic pain would occur after vaginal delivery and cesarean section. Chronic pain after delivery has not been investigated until recently. This article explores the issue of chronic pain in obstetrics.

PATHOPHYSIOLOGY OF PAIN

Nerve injury results in alterations in the structure and chemistry of the nerve. It also results in changes in the central nervous system, with modification in brain function.

Department of Anesthesiology and Critical Care, Hospital of the University of Pennsylvania, 3400 Spruce Street, Philadelphia, PA 19104, USA
* Corresponding author.
E-mail address: jason.walls@uphs.upenn.edu

Anesthesiology Clin 31 (2013) 505–515
http://dx.doi.org/10.1016/j.anclin.2013.06.001
1932-2275/13/$ – see front matter © 2013 Elsevier Inc. All rights reserved.

anesthesiology.theclinics.com

The International Association for the Study of Pain defines pain as "an unpleasant sensory and emotional experience associated with actual or potential tissue damage or described in terms of such damage" (**Box 1**).[6] This definition implies that pain from nerve injury comprises 2 aspects: the actual physical sensation and the accompanying emotional response. Although the physical sensation is common to all individualistic, the emotional component of the pain experience is individual. The pathophysiology of acute pain has been divided into 4 different steps: transduction, transmission, interpretation, and modulation. A change at any of these steps may result in the development of chronic pain.

Specific pain receptors in tissue are called *nociceptors*. Nociceptors are free nerve endings and are located in the skin, muscle, joints, and organs. Stimulation of these nociceptors results in the sensation of pain. The quality of the pain perceived by an individual on stimulation of nociceptors depends on the site of stimulation and the nature of the fibers transmitting the sensation. Sharp immediate pain is transmitted by the Aδ-fibers, and prolonged unpleasant burning pain is mediated through the smaller unmyelinated C fibers. Nociceptors have numerous different receptors on their surface that modulate their sensitivity to stimulation, including γ-aminobutyric acid, opiate, bradykinin, histamine, serotonin, and capsaicin.[7] Inflammation sensitizes this vast population of nociceptors, making them far more sensitive to stimulation (hyperalgesia). Hyperalgesia may be primary (felt at the site of stimulation) or secondary (felt at a site remote from the original injury). Activity of the C fibers may be upregulated peripherally by serotonin, prostaglandins, thromboxane, and leukotrienes in the damaged tissue.[8]

The gray matter of the spinal cord is divided into 10 laminae. The dorsal part is divided into 5 laminae (I–V), which deal with most incoming pain fibers. The unmyelinated C fibers are important carriers of burning pain and synapse in lamina II. Thin myelinated Aδ-fibers, which deal with more localized pain, synapse in laminae I and V. After synapsing in the dorsal horn, the pain sensation is transmitted centrally through various pathways. The spinothalamic pathway crosses the midline and ascends on the opposite side of the spinal cord to the ventral posterolateral nucleus of the thalamus. This nucleus is subdivided for a specific area of the body, with each area projecting to its own section of the primary sensory cortex. The spinoreticular pathway ascends on both sides of the spinal cord to the intralaminar nuclei of both the right and left thalamus. From there, the next neuron in the chain takes the information to the many areas of the brain, such as the anterior part of the cingulate gyrus (emotion), the amygdala (memory and emotion), and the hypothalamus (emotion and vascular response to emotion). No discrete center exists where pain is recognized in the cortex.

Pain is so important to survival that almost the whole brain is involved. Descending modulation of pain sensation originates from the cortex, thalamus, and brainstem (the periaqueductal gray matter). Descending pathways modulate incoming pain impulses. Notable neurotransmitters mediating this antinociceptive effect include

Box 1
Acute pain
Components of Acute Pain
Physical trauma to tissue
Emotional response to the physical trauma to tissue

norepinephrine, especially in the locus coeruleus, and serotonin in the raphe nuclei.[9] The centralization of pain occurs in all individuals. In those who develop chronic pain, these changes within the brain are maladaptive. Centralization refers to the process in which brain changes that are initially driven by nociception become maladaptive and continue to be activated.[10]

RISK FACTORS FOR CHRONIC PAIN

The uncertainty in the pathophysiology of pain is the reason that some individuals continue to have central activation despite the absence of nociceptor activation. These individuals are the ones who develop chronic pain. Several factors increase the risk of chronic pain development, such as age, gender, genetics, and preexisting pain (**Box 2**). Chronic pain is rarely described in pediatric patients.[11] Whether this decreased incidence of occurrence is from differences in the central nervous system or whether being young provides a protective effect is unclear.

The difference in the incidence of chronic pain is best exemplified by examining the incidence of chronic pain after inguinal hernia repair or thoracotomy. For inguinal hernia repair, one study showed that the incidence of chronic pain in the pediatric population is 2% for moderate pain, and that pain occurs mainly during sports activities.[12] That incidence is markedly less than the 20% incidence reported in adults. This study further investigated whether having the surgery at a very young age affected the incidence of chronic pain. No difference was seen in the incidence or severity of chronic pain if the hernia was repaired before 3 months of age compared with after 3 months of age. A recent survey of 98 children receiving inguinal hernia repair[13] (average age of respondents, 4.8 years) also showed a lower incidence of chronic pain than that seen in the adult population (5.1% vs 20.0%, respectively).

The lower incidence of chronic pain in children also occurs with other surgical procedures. Of 88 patients undergoing thoracotomy (average age of patients, 39.3 years), 14 had pain lasting greater than 3 months.[14] An inverse correlation was seen between the development of chronic pain and age of the patient at the time of surgery. Younger age resulted in a lower risk of developing chronic pain.

Gender also affects the risk of developing chronic pain after surgery. Women report greater pain after surgical procedures compared with men, and the incidence of chronic pain in women is double that of men.[15]

Genetics also plays a role in the development of chronic pain. Pain-related gene candidates include polymorphisms of catechol-O-methyltransferase, genetic variants of voltage-gated sodium channels, guanosine 5'-triphosphate cyclohydrolase,

---

Box 2
Risk factors for chronic pain

Female sex

Adult versus pediatric patient

Smoking

Type of surgery: open versus laparoscopic

Pain before procedure

Genetic predisposition

Poorly managed postoperative pain

tetrahydrobiopterin-related genes, and the μ-opioid receptor.[16] Among patients undergoing cardiac surgery, Devor[17] noted a subset who developed chronic pain in the chest and the site of vein harvest. The likelihood of developing chronic pain at both sites was extremely likely in a subset of the population examined, suggesting that these patients had a genetic predisposition to the development of chronic pain. He attributed this increased likelihood to a genetic predisposition.

Certain physical factors of the patient increase the risk of chronic pain after surgery. One of the largest studies investigated postherniotomy pain in 442 patients.[13] Of these patients, 55 had moderate to severe pain 6 months after surgery. Patients with decreased preoperative activity had a greater chance of developing chronic pain. Patients who received a heat stimulus and who rated this stimulus as painful were also more likely to develop chronic pain. Both of these risk factors suggest that the patients with pain before surgery or those with a low pain threshold have a greater likelihood of developing chronic pain. This postulate has been confirmed in other studies. In another study of 84 patients receiving radical prostatectomy, those who had pain either elsewhere or in urologic body areas were more likely to develop chronic postsurgical pain.[18]

Nicotine interacts with the nicotinic acetylcholine receptor and is delivered through cigarette smoking. Nicotine has been shown to produce analgesia, with the mechanism not completely understood.[19] It is believed to activate the descending central inhibitory pain pathway. A trial of 40 patients undergoing general abdominal surgical procedures randomized half to a transdermal nicotine patch and the other half to placebo.[20] Transdermal nicotine decreased postoperative pain scores. Although it has some potential in the management of acute pain, smoking is not beneficial for treating chronic pain. Daily smokers are more likely to develop chronic pain than nonsmokers. Furthermore, stopping smoking seems to decrease the chance of developing chronic pain.[21]

The previous study examining risk factors for postherniotomy pain is important, because not all of the surgical procedures were performed in the same manner. Some of the procedures were an open hernia repair and others were laparoscopic transabdominal preperitoneal groin repair.[13] Despite having ultimately the same repair, open surgery had a greater association with chronic pain than laparoscopic procedures.

The major question concerning the development of chronic pain is whether poorly managed acute surgical pain increases the risk of developing postsurgical chronic pain. Katz and colleagues[22] followed 30 patients for 1.5 years after thoracotomy. The only predictor for the development of chronic pain was early postoperative pain. Pain intensity at 24 hours at rest and with movement was significantly higher in the individuals who developed chronic pain. The results from this study suggest that effective management of acute pain after surgery may decrease the risk of developing chronic pain.

PREVENTION OF CHRONIC PAIN

Given that intense postoperative pain increases the risk of the developing chronic postsurgical pain, many individuals have postulated that epidural anesthesia and postoperative analgesia will prevent the development of this chronic pain. Epidural anesthesia and postoperative analgesia will prevent the nociceptor activation from reaching the central nervous system. This concept is termed *preemptive analgesia*. Gottschalk and colleagues[23] randomized 100 patients undergoing radical prostatectomy to either epidural bupivacaine 0.5%, epidural fentanyl, or no epidural analgesia.

However, all patients received postoperative epidural analgesia. This study's hypothesis was that the central sensitization that occurs with surgical incision may be prevented by dense epidural blockade before surgical incision. The group who received epidural bupivacaine or fentanyl had less pain and better return to activities of daily living at 9 weeks postoperatively than the group who did not receive intraoperative epidural medication.

This result was confirmed in another study examining phantom limb pain in patients receiving amputation.[24] In this study, 24 patients were randomized to receive an epidural infusion of bupivacaine/diamorphine/clonidine or no infusion. Those in the epidural infusion group received this medication 1 to 2 days preoperatively and at least 3 days postoperatively. At 1-year follow-up, only 1 patient in the epidural infusion group had phantom limb pain compared with 8 in the non-epidural group.

A Cochrane review examining 23 studies[25] showed that epidural anesthesia may reduce the risk of developing chronic pain after thoracotomy in approximately 1 of every 4 patients treated, and that paravertebral block may reduce the risk of chronic pain after breast cancer surgery in 1 of every 5 women treated.

Although epidural anesthesia/analgesia has been postulated for preventing chronic pain, the current hypothesis is that a systemic multimodal approach to analgesia is as effective. In this approach, various pharmacologic agents are used that address different steps in the development of acute pain. Nonsteroidal anti-inflammatory drugs are nonselective inhibitors of the enzyme cyclooxygenase. Through inhibiting this enzyme, these medications prevent the formation of prostaglandins and thromboxane from arachidonic acid. Prostaglandins and thromboxane are important substances that increase the upregulation of the C fibers. Ketamine is another analgesic that has been suggested to decrease the risk of the development of chronic pain. Ketamine is an antagonist of N-methyl-D aspartate (NMDA) receptor; NMDA may be involved in the development of chronic pain. Remerand and colleagues[26] investigated the effect of ketamine on the development of chronic pain in 154 patients receiving total hip arthroplasty. In this study, patients were randomized to receive either ketamine at 0.5 mg/kg before incision with an infusion for 24 hours of 2 μg/kg/min, or saline. Three months after the procedure, only 8% of patients in the ketamine group had pain in the operated hip compared with 21% of those in the saline group.

Gabapentin was initially developed as an anticonvulsant. Gabapentin is an analog of γ-aminobutyric acid and interacts with the calcium channels in the central nervous system. Although developed as an anticonvulsant, gabapentin was found to have analgesic properties; it decreases postoperative opioid use and is effective for treating neuropathic pain. Pregabalin is structurally similar to gabapentin but is more lipophilic, resulting in greater crossing of the blood–brain barrier. Compared with gabapentin, pregabalin is more potent and is absorbed faster. Several studies have reported that gabapentin and pregabalin are effective in preventing postsurgical chronic pain. A meta-analysis that included 11 studies showed that perioperative administration of these drugs reduced the incidence of chronic postsurgical pain.[27] The binding of these medications to a subunit of the voltage-dependent calcium channel is the postulated mechanism of action.

OBSTETRIC PATIENTS

Given that risk factors for chronic pain include surgical trauma and female gender, one would expect that chronic pain would be a significant problem in the obstetric population. Obstetric patients undergo significant trauma to tissue during vaginal and cesarean delivery. Some studies suggest that the incidence of chronic pain after cesarean delivery is between 6% and 18%, whereas the incidence of chronic pain after vaginal delivery is between 4% and 10%.[28]

ACUTE PAIN IN OBSTETRICS

Labor and delivery is a painful process associated with tissue trauma and inflammatory changes experienced as part of a multidimensional perception influenced by physiologic, psychologic, and cultural factors.[28,29] In an attempt to quantify this pain, Melzack[30] asked women to rate their pain during labor and delivery and compared the values to those obtained from patients in a general pain clinic and emergency department. Only amputation of a digit exceeded the pain of labor and delivery. The sensory words these women used to describe the pain were "sharp," "cramping," "aching," "throbbing," "stabbing," "hot," "shooting," and "tight."

Although a physiologic basis exists for labor pain, it may become modified by psychological factors. Religious and philosophic theories attempt to explain peripartum pain, but clear physiologic mechanisms of pain are present during labor and vaginal delivery. The process of labor is classically divided into 3 stages. The first stage of labor begins with the onset of uterine contractions and cervical dilation and ends with complete dilation of the cervix. The second stage of labor, also known as *fetal descent*, begins with full dilation of the cervix and ends with delivery of the baby. The third stage of labor begins with delivery of the baby and ends with delivery of the placenta.

The pain resulting from the first stage of labor is primarily caused by dilation of the cervix, with consequent distention and stretching. Because the baby's head pushing against the cervix causes this dilation, the pain of the first stage only occurs as the uterus contracts, forcing the fetal head against the cervix. Although cervical dilation accounts for most of the pain, pain from uterine contraction also occurs as the pressure and stretching of the uterine muscles stimulate the high threshold mechanoreceptors. The pain is typically described as a visceral pain; a strong dull pain over the lower abdomen between the umbilicus and symphysis pubis, laterally over the iliac crest in a band-like distribution, and posteriorly in the skin and soft tissue over the lower lumbar spines. The location of this pain is explained by the innervation of the uterus and cervix and the concept of referred pain. The sensory nerves that transmit noxious impulses that produce pain from the uterus and cervix enter the spinal cord at T10, T11, T12, and L1. These sensory fibers pass from the uterus and cervix and accompany the sympathetic nerves as they pass through the cervical plexus to the hypogastric plexus to the lumbar and thoracic sympathetic chain and then through the white rami communicantes and posterior roots associated with T10–L1. These visceral afferents synapse within laminae V of the dorsal horn. All of the lamina V cells that respond to visceral high-threshold afferents also respond to low-threshold cutaneous afferents from an area of skin supplied by the same spinal cord segment. Thus, these lamina V cells, with the convergence of somatic and visceral fibers, provide the basis for referred pain, which occurs with each uterine contraction. The mother feels the pain in the abdomen, hips, and lower back rather than the uterus and cervix, because the pain is referred to these areas.

The pain resulting from the second stage of labor occurs as the fetus descends through the birth canal. This movement results in stretching and tearing of fascia, skin, subcutaneous tissue, and other somatic structures. This somatic pain is transmitted primarily through the pudendal nerve, which is derived from the anterior primary divisions of sacral nerves S2, S3, and S4. The woman knows exactly where it hurts: the perineum. The fetus often begins to descend during the first stage of labor. During the transitional stage of the first stage, the mother often experiences both visceral and somatic pain.

Compared with the pain associated with many common surgical procedures, acute pain experienced during and after vaginal delivery is nearly universally described by women as "severe" or "horrible." In fact, within 36 hours after delivery, 10.9% of women described the pain as severe, with current estimates showing that roughly 500,000 women per year in the United States experience acute pain.[31] Other studies show that 57% of women experiencing acute pain after delivery have difficulty performing daily activities, including walking and sleep, and experience depression. Overall, perineal laceration, episiotomy, and forceps delivery were associated with increased postpartum pain.[32]

Cesarean delivery involves delivery of the infant through the abdomen, and therefore is accompanied by the surgical trauma of an incision to the abdomen and stretching of the muscles. Regarding postoperative analgesia, patients recovering from cesarean section differ from those recovering from general surgery in that mothers may desire analgesia but also want minimal sedation so that they can interact with their newborn.

CHRONIC PAIN AFTER VAGINAL DELIVERY

Although tissue trauma does not necessitate the development of chronic pain, recent evidence suggests that tissue injury related to vaginal delivery specifically may increase the risk of chronic pain via 2 mechanisms. During pregnancy, the uterine cervix and lower uterine segment sprout sensory afferent fibers through estrogen signaling and transient receptor vanilloid 1 channels, sensitizing the cervix to distention. Additionally, prostaglandins and cytokines, both inflammatory mediators that influence nociceptor sensitization, are key components of cervical remodeling before labor and delivery. These 2 mechanisms suggest an increased sensitivity to aspects of pain during vaginal delivery that could lead to the development of chronic pain.[31]

However, the incidence of chronic pain after vaginal delivery is estimated to occur in only 10% of women at 2 months postpartum.[33] Although previous reports state that the incidence of persistent pain after vaginal delivery continues to be 10% at 1 year and perineal pain continues to be 5% to 33% at 1 to 2 years after delivery, recent reports find the incidence to be more rare.[32,33] A recent multicenter, prospective, longitudinal cohort of 1228 women found that the incidence of new-onset chronic pain after vaginal delivery and cesarean delivery combined was less than 2.8% and 0.9% at 6 months and 1 year, respectively. This study specifically investigated new-onset pain temporally and physically attributed to vaginal delivery, whereas previous studies did not differentiate between new chronic pain versus previous pain syndromes, including back pain and headache. Of women experiencing persistent pain, nearly 60% described constant or daily pain at 2 months. However, by 1 year most women described mild pain, with only 15% stating that pain interfered with daily activities, and 1% describing constant pain.

Risk factors for the development of chronic pain after vaginal delivery vary between studies. However, several investigations found a significant correlation between the severity of acute pain after delivery and the development of chronic postpartum pain.[31,33] In fact, current evidence suggests a 2.5-fold increased risk of chronic pain at 2 months in patients with acute pain compared with those with mild pain after vaginal delivery. Additionally, and somewhat surprising, no direct relationship was seen between the development of new chronic pain in patients with a known history of chronic pain, varying from previous reports suggesting a link between previous pain history and new persistent pain.[31] Although the development of chronic pain correlates with the severity of acute pain and each individual pain response, it does not seem to be related to the physical trauma of birth when roughly comparing cesarean section to vaginal birth. Previous evidence suggests a difference between chronic pain at 1 year after vaginal delivery compared with cesarean section; however, recent studies indicate no difference between new-onset chronic pain related to method of delivery.[33]

Although vaginal delivery provides several physiologic mechanisms for the potential development of chronic pain; persistent pain after vaginal delivery is a rare phenomenon. Future research must further characterize the incidence and risk for the development of chronic pain, and investigate any protective effects of pregnancy against the development of chronic pain.

CHRONIC PAIN AFTER CESAREAN DELIVERY

Nikolajsen and colleagues[34] were the first to investigate chronic pain after cesarean delivery. They sent a questionnaire to 244 women who underwent cesarean delivery 6 months to 1 year prior. A total of 220 patients responded, with most no longer experiencing pain within 3 months of the cesarean delivery. However, 12.3% of patients (n = 27) still complained of pain at 6 months after delivery, with 13 of these experiencing daily pain. The 2 identified risk factors for the development of chronic pain were the use of general anesthesia for the cesarean delivery (compared with spinal anesthesia) and higher pain in the postoperative period. Again, severe acute postoperative pain has been suggested to increase the risk of development of chronic pain after cesarean delivery. This hypothesis has been confirmed by others researchers. Sng and colleagues[35] investigated the incidence and risk factors for chronic pain after cesarean delivery using spinal anesthesia. In this study of 857 patients, 51 patients had persistent pain 3 months after delivery, with 5 patients having constant pain and 5 having daily pain. The largest risk factors for the development of chronic pain were higher pain scores in the immediate postoperative period and the presence of pain elsewhere.

The procedure itself increases the risk of chronic pain. For cesarean delivery, a Pfannenstiel incision is frequently used. With a Pfannenstiel incision, the surgeon cuts on a generally horizontal (slightly curved) line just above the pubic symphysis. This incision provides the best access to organs in the central pelvis and has a low incidence of incisional hernias. Patients prefer this incision because it is cosmetically pleasing; the scar will be hidden by the pubic hair and will not distort the naval. However, this incision may be associated with entrapment of the lower abdominal wall nerves, such as the iliohypogastric or ilioinguinal nerves.[36] Factors that increase the risk of chronic pain associated with this incision are emergency cesarean delivery and recurrent Pfannenstiel incision. In the women who develop chronic pain, more than half of those with moderate to severe pain have nerve entrapment.

After cesarean delivery, neuraxial morphine is frequently administered to manage postoperative pain. In a significant number of individuals, the analgesia from this neuraxial morphine is insufficient. In a study comparing intrathecal to epidural morphine in women receiving cesarean section, the intrathecal group had greater intravenous morphine requirements postoperatively.[37] However, both groups had a requirement for intravenous morphine in the postoperative period. This requirement suggests that patients were experiencing some form of pain. The management of this pain requires a multimodal approach in which a combination of several analgesics act through different mechanisms to achieve effective pain control and prevent the development of chronic pain. Medications that are effective include nonsteroidal anti-inflammatory drugs, ketamine, and local anesthetics.[38] Although several studies confirm that increased postoperative pain raises the risk of development of chronic pain, no study has proven that a multimodal approach prevents or decreases its incidence.

Several authors have reported an incidence of chronic pain after cesarean delivery of 10% to 15%.[31–33] However, this incidence was recently questioned by a study examining 1228 women who delivered vaginally and through cesarean section.[31] At 2, 6, and 12 months after delivery, the investigators contacted the women via telephone. Of the participating women, 32% delivered via cesarean delivery. Approximately 95% of all participating women had experienced pain at 36 hours. At 6 months, only 6 women who delivered via cesarean section were experiencing chronic pain. In none of these patients did the pain interfere with sleep, work, or driving. Only 1 patient experienced constant pain, and 3 patients had pain localized to the pelvis. The results of this study have 2 explanations. The first plausible explanation is that chronic pain is not an issue after cesarean delivery. The other explanation is that this group effectively managed the postoperative pain thus reducing the risk. The investigators are all experienced anesthesiologists who were aware of the importance of postoperative analgesia; they may have used a multimodal approach to the management of pain. Either supposition is possible.

SUMMARY

Chronic pain is a phenomenon that has gained recent interest in anesthesia. The perioperative management of patients seems to affect the development of chronic pain. If a patient experiences severe postoperative pain, that patient may continue to have pain 2 months after the surgical procedure. This pain has been well described after thoracotomy, mastectomy, and hernia repair. Vaginal and cesarean delivery are associated with significant trauma to the tissue, and women often experience severe postpartum pain. Cesarean delivery is the most common surgical procedure in the United States. Chronic pain occurring after vaginal or cesarean delivery would be a significant problem. Several authors have noted an incidence of 10% to 20% of chronic pain after delivery. However, a well-conducted study recently showed that the incidence of chronic pain (persisting at 2 months after delivery) and pain at 6 months after delivery is low (1%–2%).[31] This low incidence may be because pregnancy may be protective against the development of chronic pain, or because this study was conducted in major academic centers where effective multimodal analgesia was provided. Further studies will reveal which of the these 2 hypotheses is correct.

REFERENCES

1. Borsook D, Kussman BD, George E, et al. Surgically induced neuropathic pain: understanding the perioperative process. Ann Surg 2013;257:403–12.
2. Ephraim PL, Wegener ST, MacKenzie EJ, et al. Phantom pain, residual limb pain, and back pain in amputees: results of a national survey. Arch Phys Med Rehabil 2005;86:1910–9.
3. Gaertner R, Jensen MB, Nielsen J, et al. Prevalence of and factors associated with persistent pain following breast cancer surgery. JAMA 2009;302:1985–92.
4. Kalso E, Perttunen K, Kaasinen S. Pain after thoracic surgery. Acta Anaesthesiol Scand 1992;36:96–100.
5. Aasvang EK, Kehlet H. Chronic pain after childhood groin hernia repair. J Pediatr Surg 2007;42:1403–8.

6. Merskey H, Albe-Fessard DG, Bonica JJ, et al. Pain terms: a list with definitions and notes on usage. Recommended by the IASP Subcommittee on Taxonomy. Pain 1979;6:249–52.

7. Johnson Q, Borsheski RR, Reeves-Viets JL. Pain management miniseries. Part 1. A review of management of acute pain. Mo Med 2013;110:74–9.

8. Ito S, Okuda-Ashitaka E, Minarni T. Central and peripheral roles of prostaglandins in pain and their interactions with novel neuropeptides nociception and nocistatin. Neurosci Res 2001;41:299–332.

9. Heinricher MM, Tavares I, Leith JL, et al. Descending control of nociceptions: specificity, recruitment and plasticity. Brain Res Rev 2009;60:214–25.

10. Ochoa JL. Pain mechanisms in neuropathy. Curr Opin Neurol 1994;7:407–14.

11. Maguire MF, Ravenscroft A, Beggs D, et al. A questionnaire study investigating the prevalence of the neuropathic component of chronic pain after thoracic surgery. Eur J Cardiothorac Surg 2006;29:800–5.

12. Kristensen AD, Ahlburg P, Lauridsen MC, et al. Chronic pain after inguinal hernia repair in children. Br J Anaesth 2012;109:603–8.

13. Aasvang EK, Gmaehle E, Hansen JB, et al. Predictive risk factors for persistent postherniotomy pain. Anesthesiology 2010;112:957–69.

14. Kristensen AD, Pedersen TA, Hjortadal VE, et al. Chronic pain in adults after thoracotomy in childhood or youth. Br J Anaesth 2010;104:75–9.

15. Voscopoulos C, Lema M. When does acute pain become chronic? Br J Anaesth 2010;105:i69–85.

16. Grosu I, de Kock M. Pain, opioid-induced hyperalgesia, and other measures. Anesthesiol Clin 2011;29:311–27.

17. Devor M. Evidence for heritability of pain in patients with traumatic neuropathy. Pain 2004;108:200–1.

18. Gerbershagen HJ, Ozgur E, Dagtekin O, et al. Preoperative pain as a risk factor for chronic post-surgical pain – six month follow-up after radical prostatectomy. Eur J Pain 2009;13:1054–61.

19. Shi Y, Weingarten TN, Mantilla CB, et al. Smoking and pain: pathophysiology and clinical implications. Anesthesiology 2010;113:977–92.

20. Connell-Price J, Cheng S, Flood P. Transdermal nicotine patch for postoperative pain management: a pilot dose-ranging study. Anesth Analg 2008;107:1005–10.

21. Jakobsson U. Tobacco use in relation to chronic pain: results from a Swedish population survey. Pain Med 2008;9:1091–7.

22. Katz J, Jackson M, Kavanagh BP, et al. Acute pain after thoracic surgery predicts long-term post-thoracotomy pain. Clin J Pain 1996;12:50–5.

23. Gottschalk A, Smith DS, Jobes DR, et al. Preemptive epidural analgesia and recovery from radical prostatectomy: a randomized controlled trial. JAMA 1998;279:1076–82.

24. Jahangiri M, Jayatunga AP, Bradley JW, et al. Prevention of phantom limb pain after major lower limb amputation by epidural infusion of diamorphine, clonidine, and bupivacaine. Ann R Coll Surg Engl 1994;76:324–6.

25. Andreae MH, Andreae DA. Local anaesthetics and regional anaesthesia for preventing chronic pain after surgery. Cochrane Database Syst Rev 2012;(10):CD007105. http://dx.doi.org/10.1002/14651858.CD007105.pub2.

26. Remerand F, Le Tendre C, Baud A, et al. The early and delayed analgesic effects of ketamine after total hip arthroplasty: a prospective, randomized, controlled, double-blind study. Anesth Analg 2009;109:1963–71.

27. Clarke H, Bonin RP, Orser BA, et al. The prevention of chronic postsurgical pain using gabapentin and pregabalin: a combined systematic review and meta-analysis. Anesth Analg 2012;115:428–42.
28. Vermelis JM, Wassen MM, Fiddelers AA, et al. Prevalence and predictors of chronic pain after labor and delivery. Curr Opin Anaesthesiol 2010;23:295–9.
29. Flood P, Wong CA. Chronic pain secondary to childbirth: does it exist? Anesthesiology 2013;118:16–8.
30. Melzack R. The myth of painless childbirth (the John J. Bonica lecture). Pain 1984;19:321–37.
31. Eisenach JC, Pan P, Smiley RM, et al. Resolution of pain after childbirth. Anesthesiology 2013;118:143–51.
32. Eisenach JC, Pan PH, Smiley R, et al. Severity of acute pain after childbirth, but not type of delivery, predicts persistent pain and postpartum depression. Pain 2008;140:87–94.
33. Kainu JP, Sarvela J, Tiipana E, et al. Persistent pain after caesarean section and vaginal birth: a cohort study. Int J Obstet Anesth 2010;19:4–9.
34. Nikolajsen L, Soresnsen HC, Jensen TS, et al. Chronic pain following caesarean section. Acta Anaesthesiol Scand 2004;48:111–6.
35. Sng BL, Sia AT, Quek K, et al. Incidence and risk factors for chronic pain after caesarean section under spinal anaesthesia. Anaesth Intensive Care 2009;37:748–52.
36. Loos MJ, Scheltina MR, Mulders LG, et al. The Pfannenstiel incision as a source of chronic pain. Obstet Gynecol 2008;111:839–46.
37. Duale C, Frey C, Bolandard F, et al. Epidural versus intrathecal morphine for postoperative analgesia after Caesarean section. Br J Anaesth 2003;91:690–4.
38. Lavand'homme P. Postcesarean analgesia: effective strategies and association with chronic pain. Curr Opin Anaesthesiol 2006;19:244–8.

The Changing Role of Magnesium in Obstetric Practice

Wendy A. Haft, MD[a], Manuel C. Vallejo, MD, DMD[b],*

KEYWORDS

- Magnesium • Obstetric anesthesia • Preeclampsia • Eclampsia
- Antiepileptic drugs • Neuroprotection • Cerebral palsy • Tocolysis

KEY POINTS

- Magnesium sulfate is a frequently used drug in obstetric practice.
- Known applications for magnesium sulfate in obstetrics include neuroprotection in preterm labor, seizure prophylaxis and treatment of eclampsia, tocolysis, adjuvant pain management, and therapy for acute asthma exacerbations.
- Despite its numerous benefits, magnesium sulfate can be toxic when given in large doses to at-risk patients; thus care should be exercised when prescribing magnesium sulfate therapy.

CLINICAL APPLICATIONS

Neuroprotection in Preterm Labor

Over many years, anecdotal evidence has shown a relationship between maternal magnesium sulfate therapy in obstetrics and decreased neurologic morbidity in preterm infants.[1] As a result, several multicenter trials have been conducted to better evaluate this relationship.[2] Cerebral palsy is a group of chronic, debilitating neurologic disorders and the most common motor disability present in childhood. Preterm delivery is a risk factor for the development of cerebral palsy, particularly birth at or before 34 weeks' gestational age.[3]

In 1995, a case-control study by Nelson and Grether[4] showed that low-birth-weight infants exposed to magnesium sulfate in the antenatal period were less likely to develop cerebral palsy. This study prompted several multicenter, randomized control trials to help determine if magnesium sulfate has a protective role against neurologic damage in preterm infants. The Australian Collaborative Trial of Magnesium Sulfate (ACTOMgSO4) Collaborative Group compared neonatal and infant mortality and

[a] Department of Anesthesiology, UPMC, 3471 Fifth Avenue, Suite 910, Pittsburgh, PA 15213, USA; [b] Obstetric Anesthesia, Department of Anesthesiology, Magee-Womens Hospital of UPMC, 300 Halket Street, Suite 3510, Pittsburgh, PA 15213, USA
* Corresponding author.
E-mail address: vallejomc@anes.upmc.edu

Anesthesiology Clin 31 (2013) 517–528
http://dx.doi.org/10.1016/j.anclin.2013.03.002
1932-2275/13/$ – see front matter © 2013 Elsevier Inc. All rights reserved.

occurrence of cerebral palsy in offspring of women treated with magnesium sulfate versus placebo over a follow-up period of 2 years.[5] The results of this trial showed that rates of mortality, cerebral palsy, and long-term disability were lower in the infants of mothers treated with magnesium sulfate.[6] This result is in contrast to a previous study, published in 2002, which found higher rates of adverse outcomes in infants of mothers treated with magnesium for both cerebral protection and tocolysis when compared with the infants of mothers treated with a placebo.[7] However, the differences between groups found in this study, the Magnesium and Neurologic Endpoints Trial (MagNET), were not statistically significant and prompted further research investigating the safety and efficacy of magnesium sulfate use in parturients.

In 2008, results from the Beneficial Effects of Antenatal Magnesium Sulfate (BEAM) Trial were published and showed decreased rates of cerebral palsy and mortality in the infants of patients treated with magnesium as a loading dose (6 g) followed by infusion (2 g/h) when compared with parturients receiving placebo. This was a large, multicenter trial, which included 2241 patients. All of these patients were in preterm labor at less than 32 weeks' gestation. The investigators found a statistically significant decrease in the development of cerebral palsy among infants of mothers treated with magnesium sulfate compared with placebo. However, the decrease in mortality found in this study among infants born to mothers treated with magnesium sulfate was not statistically significant.[8]

The mechanism behind the ability of magnesium to prevent neurologic damage in preterm infants remains unclear. Proposed mechanisms for these neuroprotective properties include attenuation of the neurotoxic effects of calcium through inhibition of N-methyl-D-aspartic acid (NMDA) receptors, increased cerebral blood flow through its vasodilatory effects, and the action of magnesium sulfate as a scavenger of oxygen-free radicals.[5]

Several large, multicenter trials have shown that magnesium sulfate treatment in preterm labor may afford neuroprotection for infants by reducing the risk of cerebral palsy and long-term motor dysfunction. However, care should be exercised because magnesium therapy is not without risk. Overall, research on magnesium therapy for neuroprotection in preterm labor has shown that the most benefit is achieved in parturients less 34 weeks' gestational age.[9]

Preeclampsia

The use of magnesium sulfate in preeclamptic patients aims at preventing the development of seizures and progression to eclampsia. Two percent to 8% of pregnancies are complicated by preeclampsia, a disorder associated with hypertension and proteinuria.[10] Morbidity and mortality associated with preeclampsia and eclampsia are often the result of cerebral infarction and cerebral hemorrhage. The hypothesized mechanism behind prophylaxis of magnesium sulfate against progression to eclampsia involves its ability to vasodilate cerebral vessels. This action helps prevent vasospasm, subsequent ischemia, and progression to seizure activity.[11]

The Magnesium Sulfate for Prevention of Eclampsia Trial (Magpie trial) published in 2002 was a large, multicenter trial comparing magnesium sulfate therapy versus placebo in patients with known preeclampsia who were either in labor or recently delivered but still hospitalized. The primary outcomes investigated were progression to eclampsia and death of the fetus or infant before hospital discharge. Secondary outcomes included serious maternal morbidity and symptoms of magnesium sulfate toxicity and side effects.[10]

Results of the Magpie trial showed that patients randomized to the magnesium sulfate group had statistically significant lower rates of progression to eclampsia

(40 patients vs 96 patients). This decrease in the development of eclampsia was associated with a number needed to treat of 91. The group treated with magnesium sulfate also had lower rates of maternal mortality (11 vs 20 in the placebo group). However, no differences were found between the groups in the rate of maternal morbidity, such as cardiac arrest, respiratory arrest, renal failure, liver failure, and coagulopathies, or rate of infant mortality. The beneficial effect of magnesium sulfate therapy in patients with preeclampsia was shown in both mild and severe preeclampsia, whether therapy was instituted before or after delivery, and regardless of gestational age and parity. In addition, for most patients (84%) who did progress to eclampsia, independent of allocation, magnesium sulfate therapy was instituted at the time of their first seizure, and the authors suggest that magnesium sulfate should be first-line therapy for treatment of seizures in eclamptic patients.[10]

In addition to the cerebral effects of preeclampsia, the disease state is associated with overall increased systemic vascular resistance, increased ventricular afterload, and resultant decreased cardiac output. A persistent state of increased afterload during pregnancy in patients with preeclampsia increases the risk of prolonged left ventricular hypertrophy and overall left ventricular dysfunction.[12] Magnesium sulfate, a potent systemic vasodilator, has been shown to decrease mean arterial pressure, increase the time for diastolic filling through its negative inotropic effects, and increase cardiac index.[13] The cause of increased systemic vascular resistance in preeclamptic patients at the cellular level has been postulated to be the result of decreased synthesis of nitric oxide, which likely results in vasoconstriction and overall endothelial dysfunction.[12] Magnesium has been shown to improve endothelial function through multiple mechanisms, including calcium inhibition, attenuation of endothelial damage by oxygen-free radicals, and potentiation of endogenous vasodilators like prostaglandins and adenosine.[14]

Coates and colleagues[12] used an animal model of preeclampsia to evaluate the cardiac effects of magnesium sulfate therapy. In this study, pregnant rats were treated with N^G-nitro-L-arginine methyl ester (L-NAME), a nitric oxide synthase inhibitor, to produce a condition similar to preeclampsia characterized by hypertension and left ventricular dysfunction. The rats were allocated to 1 of 3 groups, saline, L-NAME alone, or L-NAME plus magnesium sulfate. Results showed that the rats treated with L-NAME plus magnesium sulfate, when compared with the rats treated with L-NAME alone, had increased stroke volume, increased cardiac output, and improved aortic flow. Although this study has limitations, including a small sample size and ex vivo evaluation of the hearts, it does provide insight into the potential physiology of preeclampsia and the effects of magnesium sulfate therapy.

The benefit of magnesium sulfate therapy in patients with preeclampsia seems to be multifactorial, involving both neurologic and cardiovascular mechanisms. Such benefits include the prevention of cerebral vasodilation and subsequent progression to eclampsia, as well as the attenuation of systemic vascular resistance and overall left ventricular dysfunction.

Eclampsia

Many studies have shown that magnesium sulfate can help decrease the risk of seizure development and progression to eclampsia in patients with preeclampsia. Likewise, there is evidence that magnesium acts as an effective anticonvulsant in patients with eclampsia and has been shown to more effectively reduce the risk of recurrent seizures when compared with other anticonvulsant therapies.[15]

When compared with other traditionally used anticonvulsants, such as phenytoin (Dilantin, Di-Phen, Phenytek) and diazepam (Valium), magnesium sulfate therapy is associated with a lower risk of seizure recurrence.[16] In 2010, the Cochrane Pregnancy and Childbirth Group published a review of trials comparing the efficacy of phenytoin versus magnesium therapy.[15] All trials were randomized controlled trials investigating differences in outcomes between intravenous (IV) or intramuscular (IM) magnesium and phenytoin therapy in patients diagnosed with eclampsia. Results of this review show that magnesium sulfate therapy resulted in statistically significant decreases in seizure recurrence, maternal rates of pneumonia, and intensive care unit admission when compared with phenytoin. In addition, infants born to mothers treated with magnesium sulfate had improved outcomes. Magnesium therapy is more effective than phenytoin in preventing eclamptic seizures and should be the first-line treatment in patients with eclampsia.[15]

A similar review by the Cochrane Pregnancy and Childbirth Group compared magnesium sulfate therapy and diazepam in patients with eclampsia. The results of this review show that magnesium sulfate resulted in lowers rates of seizure recurrence and maternal mortality. This review did not show significant differences in perinatal or neonatal mortality, but did show that the infants of mothers treated with magnesium sulfate were less likely to have 1-minute Apgar scores less than 7 and to remain in the hospital for more than 7 days.[17]

The mechanism behind the anticonvulsant effect of magnesium is likely related to NMDA receptor antagonism and subsequent calcium inhibition. The ability of magnesium sulfate to dilate cerebral vessels and reverse some of the endothelial injury associated with preeclampsia and eclampsia may explain the enhanced anticonvulsant effect of magnesium sulfate therapy in such patients.[18]

Tocolysis

The efficacy of magnesium sulfate for seizure prophylaxis in preeclamptic patients is well studied and most members of the obstetric community accept its use for this purpose. However, although magnesium sulfate remains one of the most commonly used tocolytic agents, controversy exists regarding this purpose. Many studies have found that magnesium sulfate is effective in delaying labor when compared with other commonly used tocolytic agents, whereas other studies bring into question both the safety and efficacy of this commonly used drug.[19]

The tocolytic effect of magnesium sulfate is caused by its reduction of uterine contractions through the blockage of calcium release and the inhibition of interactions between actin and myosin.[20] Several other tocolytics are available, including calcium channel blockers, β-mimetics, and nitroglycerine. These alternative medications also work through smooth muscle relaxation. Many of these medications have not been shown to be more effective than magnesium sulfate. However, many argue that the other available tocolytics have less associated toxicity and result in lower maternal and fetal morbidity and mortality.[21]

An analysis by the Cochrane Pregnancy and Childbirth Group published in 2009 reviewed randomized controlled trials comparing magnesium sulfate therapy with placebo or alternative tocolytics for the prevention of preterm labor. Outcomes measured included efficacy of tocolysis and complications. The results of this analysis showed that patients treated with magnesium sulfate overall had no benefit in the prevention of preterm labor when compared with placebo or alternative agents. In addition, neonates and infants treated with magnesium sulfate had higher rates of morbidity and mortality. Based on these results the Cochrane Pregnancy and Childbirth Group recommends against the use of magnesium sulfate for tocolysis.[22]

However, many other studies have failed to show significant fetal or maternal morbidity and mortality when magnesium sulfate is given in low doses and for short periods. Likewise, some studies have failed to show improved efficacy among alternative tocolytics.[20] A randomized controlled trial comparing magnesium sulfate with nifedipine (Adalat, Afeditab, Nifediac, Nifedical, Procardia) showed that the group treated with magnesium sulfate was significantly less likely to deliver in the first 48 hours after the start of therapy when compared with the group treated with nifedipine. The parturients treated with magnesium sulfate were also more likely to maintain uterine quiescence during those 48 hours; however, the nifedipine group achieved uterine quiescence more quickly. The study also showed that neonates and infants exposed to magnesium sulfate were not at increased risk of morbidity and mortality. The magnesium sulfate and nifedipine groups had similar gestational ages at delivery, birth weights, and rates of admission to the intensive care unit; however, the group treated with magnesium sulfate had significantly longer lengths of stay in the intensive care unit. When evaluating for maternal adverse outcomes, significantly more parturients exposed to magnesium sulfate experienced adverse events when compared with the nifedipine group.[19]

Much controversy exists regarding the usefulness of magnesium sulfate for tocolysis. Many experts agree that magnesium sulfate therapy is most appropriate for short-term tocolysis to allow time for the institution of corticosteroid therapy and treatment of reversible causes of preterm labor. However, numerous recent studies have also shown a neuroprotective effect of magnesium sulfate in preterm labor and have found reduced rates of gross motor dysfunction and cerebral palsy in the offspring of mothers treated with magnesium sulfate. If magnesium sulfate is used, whether for the purpose of tocolysis or neuroprotection, the lowest effective dose should be used and parturients should be monitored closely for signs and symptoms of toxicity.[20]

Pain Management

The use of magnesium sulfate as an adjuvant agent for perioperative pain management is well documented.[23] Practitioners noted that patients treated with magnesium sulfate for tocolysis or preeclampsia had less pain and required fewer analgesics after cesarean section, and retrospective analysis confirmed this possible benefit.[24] NMDA receptor blockade by magnesium is the proposed mechanism for its analgesic properties through inhibition of central nociceptive stimulation. The use of magnesium sulfate as an adjuvant analgesic may be particularly useful in obstetrics, given limitations in the use of commonly used anesthetic agents, such as opioids and volatile anesthetics, because of potential for uterine atony and respiratory depression. Obstetric patients are at particular risk for awareness during cesarean section during general anesthesia as a result of avoidance of these agents, and thus, the addition of magnesium sulfate therapy may be beneficial for decreasing anesthetic requirements and the risk of intraoperative awareness.[23]

In a 2009 study in the *British Journal of Anesthesia*, parturients undergoing cesarean section were allocated to receive either saline or magnesium sulfate bolus followed by continuous infusion. Bispectral index (BIS) values were maintained between 40 and 60, with supplemental midazolam given as needed. BIS values, mean arterial pressure, total midazolam dose, total fentanyl dose, and total atracurium dose were compared between groups. The magnesium sulfate group had lower BIS values throughout surgery and reduced fentanyl, midazolam, and atracurium requirements. In addition, mean arterial pressure was found to be attenuated in parturients receiving magnesium sulfate compared with those receiving placebo.[23] However, it is possible that the vasodilatory properties of magnesium sulfate may have resulted in decreased blood pressure in this study rather than its nociceptive properties.

A double-blinded placebo-controlled trial by Paech and colleagues[24] also aimed to determine if magnesium sulfate serves as an adjuvant analgesic agent in women undergoing elective cesarean section. Patients were randomized to 1 of 3 groups, a placebo group, a high-dose magnesium group, or a low-dose magnesium group. A loading dose was given 1 hour before cesarean section and infusion immediately started and continued for 24 hours after delivery. The investigators evaluated cumulative opioid requirements over the first 48 hours of hospitalization, pain scores, overall satisfaction with pain control, time to ambulation, and time to discharge among the groups. The results showed that there was no difference in total opioid requirements at 6, 12, 24, or 48 hours among all 3 groups. Similarly, there was no difference in pain scores or patient satisfaction among the groups. The only statistically significant difference among groups was that the patients who received either high-dose or low-dose magnesium had greater blood loss than the placebo group, as estimated by the surgery team. This situation may be caused by uterine atony in the postoperative period as a result of the smooth muscle relaxant effects of magnesium sulfate.[24]

There is evidence that intrathecal magnesium sulfate may potentiate the analgesic properties of intrathecal opioids in parturients. One trial investigating this effect[25] randomized patients undergoing combined spinal epidural (CSE) to 25 μg of fentanyl with 3 mL (mL) of saline or to 25 μg of fentanyl with 50 mg of magnesium sulfate (also 3 mL). Time to first request for additional analgesia was used to define the length of analgesia provided by the intrathecal combinations. The investigators found that the patients who received magnesium with fentanyl had longer duration of analgesia, measured by longer time to first request for additional analgesic agents. This difference was 75 minutes versus 60 minutes. There was no difference found between groups in visual analog scale, motor blockade, sensory level achieved, or adverse outcomes. In another study investigating IV magnesium sulfate versus IV saline placebo added to intrathecal fentanyl during CSE,[26] no differences in the duration of analgesia were found between groups.

Overall, data are limited regarding the use of magnesium sulfate for the sole purpose of adjuvant analgesia in obstetric practice. Care should be exercised in the use of magnesium sulfate for analgesia because of the potential for adverse side effects.

Asthma

Magnesium sulfate, a smooth muscle relaxant and bronchodilator, has been studied for use in acute asthma attacks. Overall, results have been mixed, with some studies showing benefits for adults with severe asthma and others showing no effect. One study, using a 2-g IV bolus dose of magnesium sulfate, in addition to standard bronchodilator and steroid therapy, showed increased FEV_1 (forced expiratory volume in first second of expiration) and decreased hospital admission for the patients randomized to receive magnesium sulfate versus placebo.[27]

In a 2002 multicenter randomized controlled trial, investigators randomized patients to 1 of 2 groups, 2 g IV magnesium sulfate with nebulized albuterol and IV methylprednisolone or placebo with the same albuterol and methylprednisolone regimen. Patients were treated with magnesium sulfate or placebo 30 minutes after arrival at the emergency department. The primary outcome investigated was FEV_1 at 240 minutes (4 hours) after arrival. The results showed that magnesium sulfate had benefit in patients with an initial FEV_1 of less than 25% of predicted, indicating severe asthma on arrival at the emergency department. In patients with initial FEV_1 greater than 25% of predicted, no difference was found between the magnesium sulfate group and the placebo group. This study confirms the results of previous studies indicating that magnesium sulfate may be of particular benefit in patients with severe asthma.[27]

The Cochrane Group performed a review of literature investigating the benefit of nebulized magnesium sulfate in treating asthma attacks. The studies included in the review compared nebulized magnesium sulfate alone with nebulized β-agonist alone or nebulized magnesium sulfate with nebulized β-agonist with nebulized β-agonist alone. Both adult and pediatric populations were included. The results showed overall improvement in pulmonary function tests in patients treated with nebulized magnesium along with nebulized β-agonist, but this combination was statistically significant only in patients with severe asthma.[28]

There is a paucity of studies investigating the use of magnesium sulfate specifically for asthma exacerbation in pregnancy. During pregnancy, some patients with asthma experience improvement of their symptoms, whereas others have no change or worsening of their asthma symptoms. During pregnancy, increased circulating estrogen, progesterone, and prostaglandins may result in enhanced bronchodilation and improvement of asthma symptoms. However, the decreased functional residual capacity inherent in pregnancy results in atelectasis, ventilation-perfusion mismatching, and subsequent worsening of symptoms. Studies have also shown that poorly controlled asthma during pregnancy results in increased maternal and neonatal adverse events.[29] Most common asthma rescue agents have been shown to be safe for use in pregnancy, including magnesium sulfate.

Overall, data indicate that IV or nebulized magnesium sulfate therapy may be beneficial in patients with severe asthma presenting with an exacerbation. Most studies also show that magnesium sulfate is most effective when combined with mainstay treatments such as β-agonist therapy and corticosteroids and in patients suffering from severe asthma.

DOSING

Magnesium sulfate is generally given as an IV bolus followed by continuous infusion for many indications, including seizure prophylaxis in preeclampsia and eclampsia, tocolysis, neuroprotection in preterm labor, and pain management. There are often wide ranges in recommendations for dosage for such indications. Given the serious risks associated with magnesium sulfate toxicity, conservative treatment regimens should be followed with use of the lowest possible effective dose.[9] For most indications, the continuous infusion typically continues for no more than 24 hours.[10] It is suggested that serum concentrations of magnesium range from 2 to 4 mmol/L. However, studies have suggested that monitoring of patellar reflexes and respiratory rate is more beneficial than following serum concentration of magnesium.[1] **Table 1** indicates recommended dose ranges of magnesium for various indications.

ADMINISTRATION

For most indications, magnesium sulfate is given as an IV or IM dose.[11] In the Magpie trial, which investigated the use of magnesium sulfate in preeclampsia, it was noted that centers that used IM dosing rather than IV dosing had higher rates of progression to eclampsia and infant death.[10] Thus, some experts recommend IV dosing, particularly for this indication. Magnesium also may be given intrathecally for use as an adjuvant to intrathecal opioids and local anesthetics, with some conflicting results as to its efficacy.[25] In addition, nebulized magnesium has been studied for use in severe

Table 1
Recommended dose ranges of magnesium sulfate according to indication

Indication	Loading Dose	Continuous Infusion	Alternative Dosing
Neuroprotection in preterm labor	4 g IV over 20 min[9]	1–2 g/h IV[9]	
Preeclampsia	4 g IV over 20 min[10]	1 g/h IV[10]	Per the Magpie trial: IM dosing was 5 g bolus into each buttock followed by 5 g IM every 4 h for 24 h[10]
Eclampsia	4–6 g IV over 20 min[11]	1–2 g/h IV[11]	10 g IM in divided doses in each buttock followed by 5 g IM every 4 h for 24 h[11]
Tocolysis	4 g IV over 20 min with additional boluses of 2 g IV as needed for persistent labor[19,30]	Initial infusion rate of 2 g/h IV with increase to maximum of 4 g/h IV for persistent contractions[19,30]	
Pain management	4 g IV over 20 min[26]	2 g/h IV[26]	50 mg intrathecally during spinal anesthesia[25]
Asthma	2 g IV bolus over 20 min[27]		125–500 mg nebulized; generally given as 3 doses at least 20 min apart[31]

asthma exacerbations and found to be effective when combined with nebulized β-agonists.[28]

SIDE EFFECTS

Magnesium sulfate can have life-threatening side effects when overdosed. This situation is particularly problematic given its narrow therapeutic range. It has been suggested that target serum concentrations range from 2 to 4 mmol/L; however, it has also been shown that side effects begin to appear at serum concentrations of 5 to 7 mmol/L. Adequate renal function is also necessary in any patient receiving magnesium sulfate, because it is excreted through the kidneys. For all of these reasons, the patient should be closely monitored while receiving boluses and continuous infusions of magnesium. It is particularly important that patellar reflexes, respiratory rate, serum creatinine, serum magnesium concentration, and urine output be frequently monitored.[1]

The same mechanisms responsible for the desirable clinical effects of magnesium sulfate, including vasodilation and smooth muscle relaxation, are also implicated as the cause of the undesirable side effects of magnesium sulfate. These side effects include muscle weakness, respiratory depression, and increased blood loss.[24]

Therapeutic doses of magnesium sulfate depress hyperreflexia and seizure activity through its actions at the neuromuscular junction. However, toxic doses can result in profound muscle weakness, hyporeflexia, respiratory arrest, and paralysis.[32] The inherent smooth muscle relaxant effects of magnesium sulfate, exploited in its use as a tocolytic, may result in persistent uterine atony and may increase blood loss during cesarean delivery.[24]

DRUG-DRUG INTERACTION

Magnesium sulfate has been shown to interact with several other pharmacologic agents that may be used in obstetric practice.

Neuromuscular Blocking Agents

Magnesium sulfate has been shown to potentiate the effects of neuromuscular blocking agents. Muscle weakness found with excessive doses of magnesium sulfate is believed to be caused by decreased acetylcholine release and decreased muscle fiber excitability. The same mechanisms result in the ability of magnesium sulfate to decrease hyperreflexia and seizure activity during eclampsia. It is recommended that doses of neuromuscular blocking agents be adjusted in patients receiving magnesium to avoid prolonged paralysis.[32]

Diuretics

Although thiazide and loop diuretics may result in magnesium depletion, potassium-sparing diuretics may cause hypermagnesemia by decreasing renal excretion of magnesium. Thus, combining potassium-sparing diuretics with magnesium sulfate increases the likelihood of magnesium toxicity, and so magnesium levels and signs of hypermagnesemia should be closely followed.[33]

Antibiotics

Concomitant administration of quinolones and magnesium has been shown to result in decreased absorption of this class of antibiotics.[34] Because of concerns regarding the link between fetal musculoskeletal anomalies and use of quinolones in pregnancy, quinolones are not commonly used during pregnancy; however, there is limited clinical evidence of their teratogenicity.[35]

Antihypertensives

Magnesium sulfate therapy results in decreased mean arterial pressure through both the antiadrenergic effects of calcium antagonism and decreased peripheral vascular resistance.[1] Magnesium sulfate decreases the release of catecholamines from the adrenals, and has been shown to improve hemodynamic stability in patients with pheochromocytomas.[36] Care should be exercised when combining magnesium sulfate and antihypertensive medication, because this combination may result in excessive hypotension, particularly with calcium channel blockers. However, when magnesium sulfate was compared with nitroglycerin, magnesium was found to not only be more effective as a tocolytic but also result in lower incidence of hypotensive episodes.[30]

SUMMARY

Magnesium sulfate is a frequently encountered drug in obstetric practice and has been shown to be beneficial in many clinical situations. Several recent studies have shown that magnesium sulfate may be neuroprotective by reducing cerebral palsy in preterm infants, particularly in infants born before 34 weeks' gestation.[3] There are many theories to explain the neuroprotective effects of magnesium, including inhibition at NMDA receptors, vasodilation of cerebral blood vessels, and scavenging of oxygen-free radicals.[5]

The vasodilatory effects of magnesium sulfate make it an effective therapy in pre-eclampsia, a disorder accompanied by dysfunctional endothelium and increased systemic vascular resistance.[12] Magnesium sulfate has also been shown to inhibit progression to eclampsia and to effectively reduce the recurrence of seizures in patient with eclampsia.[15]

Magnesium sulfate acts as an effective tocolytic through its ability to induce uterine atony through smooth muscle relaxation.[20] It has been shown to be more effective than other tocolytics, including nifedipine and nitroglycerin, but is also associated with more adverse maternal events.[21] Smooth muscle relaxation also results in the bronchodilating effect found with both IV and nebulized magnesium sulfate. Magnesium sulfate treatment has been shown to be most effective when combined with nebulized β-agonists and in patients with severe asthma.[28]

Magnesium sulfate may have analgesic properties through NMDA receptor inhibition.[23] Overall, data are limited regarding the use of magnesium as an analgesic during labor and delivery; however, there is evidence that addition of intrathecal magnesium sulfate to a spinal anesthetic may result in prolongation of analgesia.[25]

For most indications, magnesium sulfate is given as an initial loading dose followed by a continuous infusion. Magnesium sulfate toxicity is associated with life-threatening effects, including muscle weakness, respiratory arrest, hypotension, and uterine atony.[9] As a result, reflexes, respiratory rate, and magnesium levels should be closely followed in parturients on magnesium sulfate, and the lowest effective dose should always be used.[1]

Magnesium has been used medicinally for hundreds of years, as shown in the documentation of the use of Epsom salts as early as the seventeenth century. Magnesium sulfate was even used specifically for preeclampsia and eclampsia in the early 1900s.[1] Use of magnesium sulfate has expanded in recent years as a result of ongoing research investigating its benefits for neuroprotection in preterm labor, tocolysis, and adjuvant pain control. When carefully used, magnesium sulfate has proved to be a versatile drug with numerous benefits in the obstetric population.

REFERENCES

1. Fawcett WJ, Haxby EJ, Male DA. Magnesium: physiology and pharmacology. Br J Anaesth 1999;83(2):302–20.
2. Cahill AG, Caughey AB. Magnesium for neuroprophylaxis: fact or fiction? Am J Obstet Gynecol 2009;200(6):590–4.
3. Conde-Agudelo A, Romero R. Antenatal magnesium sulfate for the prevention of cerebral palsy in preterm infants less than 34 weeks' gestation: a systematic review and meta-analysis. Am J Obstet Gynecol 2009;200(6):595–609.
4. Nelson KB, Grether JK. Can magnesium sulfate reduce the risk of cerebral palsy in very low birthweight infants? Pediatrics 1995;95(2):263–9.
5. Cahill AG, Odibo AO, Stout MJ, et al. Magnesium sulfate therapy for the prevention of cerebral palsy in preterm infants: a decision-analytic and economic analysis. Am J Obstet Gynecol 2011;205(6):542.e1–7.
6. Crowther CA, Hiller JE, Doyle LW, et al. Effect of magnesium sulfate given for neuroprotection before preterm birth: a randomized controlled trial. JAMA 2003;290(20):2669–76.
7. Mittendorf R, Dambrosia J, Pryde PG, et al. Association between the use of antenatal magnesium sulfate in preterm labor and adverse health outcomes in infants. Am J Obstet Gynecol 2002;186(6):1111–8.

8. Rouse DJ, Hirtz DG, Thom E, et al. A randomized, controlled trial of magnesium sulfate for the prevention of cerebral palsy. N Engl J Med 2008;359(9):895–905.

9. Doyle LW, Crowther CA, Middleton P, et al. Magnesium sulphate for women at risk of preterm birth for neuroprotection of the fetus. Cochrane Database Syst Rev 2009;(1):CD004661.

10. Magpie Trial Collaborative Group. Do women with pre-eclampsia, and their babies, benefit from magnesium sulphate? The Magpie Trial: a randomised placebo-controlled trial. Lancet 2002;359:1877–90.

11. Belfort MA, Anthony J, Saade GR, et al. A comparison of magnesium sulfate and nimodipine for the prevention of eclampsia. N Engl J Med 2003;348(4):304–11.

12. Coates BJ, Broderick TL, Batia LM, et al. MgSO4 prevents left ventricular dysfunction in an animal model of preeclampsia. Am J Obstet Gynecol 2006; 195(5):1398–403.

13. Scardo JA, Hogg BB, Newman RB. Favorable hemodynamic effects of magnesium sulfate in preeclampsia. Am J Obstet Gynecol 1995;173(4):1249–53.

14. Shechter M, Sharir M, Labrador MJ, et al. Oral magnesium therapy improves endothelial function in patients with coronary artery disease. Circulation 2000; 102(19):2353–8.

15. Duley L, Henderson-Smart DJ, Chou D, et al. Magnesium sulphate versus phenytoin for eclampsia. Cochrane Database Syst Rev 2010;(10):CD000128.

16. The Eclampsia Trial Collaborative Group. Which anticonvulsants for women with eclampsia? Evidence from the Collaborative Eclampsia Trial. Lancet 1995;345: 1455–63.

17. Duley L, Henderson-Smart DJ, Walker GJ, et al. Magnesium sulphate versus diazepam for eclampsia. Cochrane Database Syst Rev 2010;(12):CD000127.

18. Pryde PG, Mittendorf R. Contemporary usage of obstetric magnesium sulfate: indication, contraindication, and relevance of dose. Obstet Gynecol 2009; 114(3):669–73.

19. Lyell DJ, Pullen K, Campbell L, et al. Magnesium sulfate compared with nifedipine for acute tocolysis of preterm labor: a randomized controlled trial. Obstet Gynecol 2007;110(1):61–7.

20. Mercer BM, Merlino AA. Magnesium sulfate for preterm labor and preterm birth. Obstet Gynecol 2009;114(3):650–68.

21. Grimes DA, Nanda K. Magnesium sulfate tocolysis: time to quit. Obstet Gynecol 2006;108(4):986–9.

22. Crowther CA, Hiller JE, Doyle LW. Magnesium sulphate for preventing preterm birth in threatened preterm labour. Cochrane Database Syst Rev 2002;(4): CD001060.

23. Lee DH, Kwon IC. Magnesium sulphate has beneficial effects as an adjuvant during general anaesthesia for Caesarean section. Br J Anaesth 2009;103(6): 861–6.

24. Paech MJ, Magann EF, Doherty DA, et al. Does magnesium sulfate reduce the short- and long-term requirements for pain relief after caesarean delivery? A double-blind placebo-controlled trial. Am J Obstet Gynecol 2006;194(6): 1596–602 [discussion: 1602–3].

25. Buvanendran A, McCarthy RJ, Kroin JS, et al. Intrathecal magnesium prolongs fentanyl analgesia: a prospective, randomized, controlled trial. Anesth Analg 2002;95(3):661–6.

26. Sullivan JT, Higgins N, Toledo P, et al. The effect of intravenous magnesium therapy on the duration of intrathecal fentanyl labor analgesia. Int J Obstet Anesth 2012;21(3):212–6.

27. Silverman RA, Osborn H, Runge J, et al. IV magnesium sulfate in the treatment of acute severe asthma: a multicenter randomized controlled trial. Chest 2002; 122(2):489–97.
28. Blitz M, Blitz S, Beasely R, et al. Inhaled magnesium sulfate in the treatment of acute asthma. Cochrane Database Syst Rev 2005;(4):CD003898.
29. Schatz M. Interrelationships between asthma and pregnancy: a literature review. J Allergy Clin Immunol 1999;103(2 Pt 2):S330–6.
30. El-Sayed YY, Riley ET, Holbrook RH Jr, et al. Randomized comparison of intravenous nitroglycerin and magnesium sulfate for treatment of preterm labor. Obstet Gynecol 1999;93(1):79–83.
31. Mohammed S, Goodacre S. Intravenous and nebulised magnesium sulphate for acute asthma: systematic review and meta-analysis. Emerg Med J 2007;24(12): 823–30.
32. Sinatra RS, Philip BK, Naulty JS, et al. Prolonged neuromuscular blockade with vecuronium in a patient treated with magnesium sulfate. Anesth Analg 1985; 64(12):1220–2.
33. Nicholls MG. Interaction of diuretics and electrolytes in congestive heart failure. Am J Cardiol 1990;65(10):17E–21E [discussion 22E–3E].
34. Polk RE. Drug-drug interactions with ciprofloxacin and other fluoroquinolones. Am J Med 1989;87(5A):76S–81S.
35. Loebstein R, Addis A, Ho E, et al. Pregnancy outcome following gestational exposure to fluoroquinolones: a multicenter prospective controlled study. Antimicrobial Agents Chemother 1998;42(6):1336–9.
36. James MF, Huddle KR, Owen AD, et al. Use of magnesium sulphate in the anaesthetic management of phaeochromocytoma in pregnancy. Can J Anaesth 1988;35(2):178–82.

Use of Advanced Airway Techniques in the Pregnant Patient

Helene Finegold, MD*, Christopher A. Troianos, MD, Hersimren Basi, MD

KEYWORDS

- Obstetric airway emergencies • Difficult airway • Difficult intubation
- Airway techniques • Airway algorithms

KEY POINTS

- Pregnancy affects the maternal airway. An understanding of these physiologic changes is required for the safe management.
- The difficult airway algorithm has been adapted for the obstetric patient. This algorithm must be practiced with the entire obstetric care team to familiarize nonanesthesia providers with the management.
- Newer airway devices have been developed. These devices are only as useful as one is familiar with them. One must practice with these devices before needing them for an airway emergency.
- A difficult airway cart must be available in the obstetric suite.
- The management of the difficult airway requires a team approach. All people who work in the obstetric suite must be familiar with the management. This familiarity requires teamwork and practice through simulation.

INTRODUCTION

There have been many advances in obstetric anesthesiology, particularly with improvements in patient safety, as evidenced by the decline in maternal morbidity and mortality.[1] However, securing the maternal airway remains a challenge to anesthesiologists. A 2-year case review in the United Kingdom confirmed the incidence of failed intubation to be 1 in 224 obstetric patients.[2] These authors keenly observed that the incidence of failed intubations has not changed during the last 20 years.[2] Although airway management techniques have developed and improved the ability to secure

Disclosures: None.
Conflicts of Interest: None.
Department of Anesthesiology, Western Pennsylvania Hospital, West Penn Allegheny Health System, 4800 Friendship Avenue, Suite 451, Pittsburgh, PA 15224, USA
* Corresponding author.
E-mail address: Finegoldh@yahoo.com

Anesthesiology Clin 31 (2013) 529–543
http://dx.doi.org/10.1016/j.anclin.2013.04.002
1932-2275/13/$ – see front matter © 2013 Elsevier Inc. All rights reserved.

the difficult airway, patient characteristics have also changed during the same time. Body mass index (BMI), advanced maternal age, and Mallampati score are independent predictors for failed intubation in the obstetric suite.[2] The average age and weight of women giving birth are increasing, along with the complexity of many cases.[3] Advanced maternal age is associated with increased comorbidities, including diabetes and obesity, which may account for the increased risk of difficult airways. Most anesthesiologists who practice obstetric anesthesia are expert and confident in their regional anesthesia skills. However, these same anesthesiologists need to practice and become more confident in airway management and in using the newer airway management techniques, as they may be required to handle a true, high-stress emergency scenario with less than ideal circumstances. The rate of maternal mortality is 10-fold higher with Cesarean delivery than with vaginal delivery, suggesting that a significant number of these women die while undergoing emergent cesarean delivery requiring general anesthesia.[4] The time pressure associated with inducing general anesthesia in the obstetric patient is a significant problem. A computational simulation model used to estimate the rate of oxygen desaturation in pregnant women revealed that pregnant women with a BMI of 50 kg/m^2 will have oxygen desaturation in 90 seconds, whereas normal weight pregnant patients will tolerate approximately 3.5 minutes of apnea before significant decreases in saturation are observed.[5]

Anesthesiologists are typically well trained in the management of the difficult airway; however, obstetric patients have unique changes that make the difficult airway even more challenging. Practitioners must understand the expected changes in the maternal airway and physiology to anticipate the needs of the patient and the potential problems encountered with airway management. Hormonal changes and increased blood volume contribute to edema and friability of the upper airway.[6] Nasal congestion and reduced diameter of nasal passages are also due to hormonal changes and increased blood volume.[7] Increased nasal engorgement may affect patients' ability to breathe and leads to increased rhinitis during pregnancy.[7] The facial and laryngeal edema and engorgement of the arytenoids and vocal cords that occur during labor often necessitate the placement of a smaller tracheal tube during Cesarean section. Laryngoscopy and intubation are also more difficult to perform because of the maternal airway edema. Maternal respiratory changes with term gestation include increased minute ventilation (50%), increased oxygen consumption (20%), and decreased functional residual capacity (20%).[4] These changes lead to rapid oxygen desaturation during apnea. Increased airway closure may occur during tidal ventilation, resulting in increased ventilation/perfusion mismatch and maternal hypoxia.[7] The rapid desaturation quickly leads to hypoxia when an unexpectedly difficult airway is encountered. The supine position during intubation worsens the already reduced functional residual capacity (FRC), further compounding the hypoxia that occurs during apnea.

EVALUATION OF THE AIRWAY

It is imperative that the anesthesiologist completes a history and physical with special attention to the maternal airway on all patients in the labor suite. The first encounter with an obstetric patient is usually for regional analgesia for labor or regional anesthesia for elective cesarean section. It is critical that the anesthesiologist perform and document an airway examination during this first encounter, even if general anesthesia is not planned. In a retrospective survey of failed intubation attempts in the obstetrics ward, Quinn and Milne[2] identified that many records lacked a recorded Mallampati score or any type of airway examination. This finding suggests that practitioners are not always considering the possibility of general anesthesia, thereby missing the opportunity to identify a potential difficult intubation that would allow for the appropriate preparation. The identification of a potentially difficult airway should immediately prompt a meeting with the obstetrics team. A frank discussion should ensue and a plan should be developed to avoid emergency delivery and intubation. These discussions often conclude that early placement of regional anesthesia is desirable, whereas alternate plans for emergent delivery are made. This type of teamwork and communication is important for educating obstetricians to the clinical challenges and potential morbidity to their patient that they may not realize.

Regardless of the planned procedure, anesthesiologists must be vigilant about examining the patient's airway and other possible conditions that may complicate the course of labor, delivery, and the postpartum period. Mallampati classification, neck size and range of motion, and mouth opening must be evaluated and recorded. Thyromental distance and Mallampati classification are sensitive predictors of difficult intubation.[8] The incidence of a Mallampati class 4 airway increases during pregnancy and correlates with maternal weight gain during pregnancy.[9]

Another aspect to this population is that the onset of labor is often spontaneous and the patient has not made preparation for arriving at the hospital with an empty stomach. It is critical to determine the last time the patient consumed food and liquids. Due to the spontaneous onset of labor, patients are often not fasting like elective surgical patients. Their hospital admission is not planned and therefore these patients may not have access or followed the usual preoperative anesthesia instructions. It is necessary to remove tongue rings and other jewelry on admission, because these items are difficult to remove and cause additional and unnecessary difficulty should intubation be required during the delivery. It is important to inquire about past surgical experiences and determine if the patient has a history of difficult intubation. A brief screening should be performed on all patients, even before anesthesia services are requested. It is helpful to educate nonanesthesia personnel to recognize certain risk factors on admission that should automatically trigger an anesthesia consultation. Such factors include obesity, history of anesthesia-related complications, sleep apnea, and malignant hyperthermia. This screening should trigger further investigation by the anesthesia staff and prevent last minute surprises during unexpected emergency situations. It is also important to be alerted if there is a patient with any significant comorbidities, including diabetes, obesity, or cardiac issues. Old records should be obtained regardless of the planned delivery method and kept with the patient's chart throughout the course of labor.

AIRWAY ASSESSMENT

The examination of the airway entails documenting those physical findings that predict the ability to manage the airway, including Mallampati classification, neck circumference and extension, and thyromental distance. The Mallampati classification is based on the relationship of the oral pharyngeal structures and the base of the tongue. Based on this relationship, the classification system predicts the difficulty in performing laryngoscopy successfully. Mallampati hypothesized that when the base of the tongue is disproportionately large in relation to the oropharyngeal cavity, the base of the tongue will obscure the visibility of the tonsillar pillars and the uvula, making laryngoscopy and intubation difficult.[10] There are 4 classes of in the Mallampati classification, which was further modified by Samsoon and Young[11]:

Class I: visualization of soft palate, uvula, and tonsillar pillars
Class II: visualization of soft palate and base of uvula
Class III: visualization of soft palate only
Class IV: visualization of hard palate only

Cormack and LeHane developed a grading system to classify the view of the glottic opening during laryngoscopy[12]:

Grade I: most of glottis visible
Grade II: only posterior portion of glottis visible
Grade III: only epiglottis visible
Grade IV: epiglottis not visible

Using these 2 grading systems, the difficulty of laryngoscopy and intubation can be predicted. Patients with a Mallampati score of I or II are usually not difficult to manage. Patients with a Mallampati class III and IV are often more difficult to manage and lead to a Cormack LeHane grade III and IV view.

Neck circumference and extension are also important factors to assess when evaluating the airway. Neck circumference is measured at the level of the cricoid cartilage. Neck circumference greater than 43 cm is associated with increased difficulty and failed intubation attempts.[13] Increased neck circumference is associated with obesity and increased soft tissue. Increased tissue is thought to contribute to more difficulty in obtaining a view of the glottic opening to facilitate intubation. The thyromental distance is measured from the top of the chin to the level of the thyroid cartilage in the neck. A distance greater than 6.5 cm with no other anatomic abnormalities is predictive of an easier intubation; however, a distance of less than 6 cm usually predicts a difficult intubation.[10] Neck circumference and Mallampati classification have been shown to be independent predictors for difficult intubation in obese patients.[13] Neck extension is important to align the oral, pharyngeal, and laryngeal axes during laryngoscopy. If a patient has decreased neck extension, it may compromise the ability to obtain the alignment needed for visualization. When a patient has decreased neck extension, the situation can be improved by putting the patient in the sniffing position. Using shoulder rolls and properly placed pillows, one optimizes the situation and better aligns the axes to facilitate intubation.

Key Points of Airway Examination

- Mallampoti classification
- Removal of tongue jewelry
- Assess neck mobility
- Neck circumference
- Inspection of dentition
- Thyromental distance

Aspiration is a complication of maternal airway manipulation. According to the Obstetric Anesthesia Practice Guidelines, the intake of clear liquids during labor does not increase the risk of maternal aspiration and increases maternal satisfaction.[14] Although the guidelines do not suggest specific fasting times, it is known that the ingestion of solids before operative delivery increases the risk of maternal complications. The guidelines further suggest that those patients at increased risk for difficult intubation or complications during delivery should restrict oral intake. There are many reasons that the parturient is at increased risk for aspiration. The physiologic effects of progesterone lead to smooth muscle relaxation in the gastrointestinal tract. In addition, the gravid uterus displaces the stomach upward, which changes the angle of the gastroesophageal junction.[10] Pregnancy affects the lower esophageal sphincter and this makes the parturient prone to heartburn and reflux. A nonparticulate antacid is administered before operative procedures, while rapid sequence induction with the application of cricoid pressure is recommended during the induction of general anesthesia. The increased risk of aspiration during emergent surgery is makes effective and efficient management of the airway crucial to successful outcome, as these patients have a higher probability of morbidity and mortality.

The risk of failed intubation is increased in the obese pregnant patient. Normal body weight is a BMI of 18.5 to 24.9 kg/m^2; overweight is defined as 25 to 29.9 kg/m^2 and obesity is more than 30 kg/m^2. The Confidential Enquiry into Maternal and Child Health reported that during the period of 2000 to 2002, 30% of all mothers were obese. By 2003 to 2005, more than 50% were obese or super morbidly obese.[8] As previously mentioned, there is a significantly higher risk of failed or difficult intubation associated with obesity in pregnancy. Whether the obese pregnant patient has a higher risk for aspiration versus the nonobese pregnant patient remains controversial. Obese patients have a higher incidence of hiatal hernia, gastroesophageal reflux, and elevated intragastric pressure compared with normal weight pregnant women.[8] Pregnancy will increase the development of sleep-associated breathing disorders and worsen symptoms in those with obstructive sleep apnea.[7] Obstructive sleep apnea is associated with difficult mask ventilation and hypoxia. When the obese pregnant patient is in the supine position, decreases in FRC are more exaggerated and leads to FRC falling below closing capacity, which leads to airway closure and shunting. All of these factors cause the obese pregnant patient to become hypoxemic very rapidly during apnea with induction of general anesthesia in the delivery room. Hypoxia further stresses the already depressed fetus and the tense situation in the labor room becomes even more stressful. It is even difficult to coordinate teamwork and work efficiently to care for mother and her fetus during these stressful conditions.

Indications for Tracheal Intubation

Tracheal intubation is most commonly used when an obstetrician determines the need to deliver the fetus emergently from a patient without an existing regional anesthesia sufficient for surgical anesthesia. Less common reasons for tracheal intubation with general anesthesia are the elective Cesarean section or postpartum tubal ligation. Indications for general anesthesia involving Cesarean section at 13 hospitals in Australia and New Zealand included mandated immediate delivery (43%), obstetrician request (29%), failed regional block (25%), maternal request (24%), actual or potential hemodynamic disturbance (21%), coagulopathy (5.3%), sepsis (4.0%), and other reasons (15%).[3]

During the induction of general anesthesia in the supine position, the gravid uterus increases intragastric pressure, which is further increased with polyhydramnios, multiple gestations, the lithotomy position, and by the application of fundal pressure during delivery. Oral administration of sodium citrate may be of benefit to reduce the consequences of gastric aspiration by decreasing gastric acidity; however, the limited duration of action may not protect the patient during emergence from anesthesia.

Although the American Society of Anesthesiologists has standardized the approach to the difficult airway, it is important to consider how this algorithm needs to be adapted for the obstetric patient.[15] Although there are no evidence-based guidelines for management of the obstetric difficult airway or failed obstetric intubation, there are several difficult and failed obstetric airway algorithms that are complicated because they aim to cover all contingencies.[6,16–18] Newer algorithms developed for unanticipated difficult airway in obstetrics have been used to evaluate the ability of trainees to manage 6 generic clinical situations. These situations include the clinical dilemma of "can and cannot ventilate" in a simulation environment with 3 clinical contexts: elective cesarean section, emergency cesarean section for fetal distress, and emergency cesarean section for maternal distress. Performance assessed through a critical skills checklist identified deficits among trainees as a tool to potentially improve overall management.[19]

Induction of General Anesthesia in the Pregnant Patient

The first step in inducing general anesthesia in the pregnant patient involves proper positioning of the patient on the operating room table. A difficult airway cart should always be in close proximity to the delivery room and multiple laryngoscope blades and sized tracheal tubes should be readily available. A Cardiff wedge should be placed underneath the patient's left hip to prevent supine hypotension syndrome. It may be helpful to place a roll underneath the patient's shoulder to allow for maximal alignment of the pharyngeal and tracheal axes. If needed, an assistant moves the patient's breasts caudally, to allow better access to the patient's head and neck. Adequate preoxygenation and denitrogenation are achieved by placing a mask strap and face mask to allow the patient to breathe 100% oxygen while the monitors are applied. Rapid sequence induction with cricoid should proceed with intravenous administration of an induction agent and muscle relaxant. Difficult airway algorithms as illustrated in **Fig. 1** guide the scenario of "cannot intubate and cannot ventilate." Cricoid pressure release and attempted mask ventilation are used if the patient becomes hypoxemic. Ventilation via facemask and/or supraglottic airway is necessary when the patient's saturation becomes less than 90%.[20] After establishing adequate oxygenation and ventilation, clinical decision-making requires communication with the surgical team. A stable maternal and fetal status affords the opportunity to awaken the patient and abort the procedure or secure the airway with the patient awake and spontaneously breathing. An unstable situation prompts the need for mask ventilation or a supraglottic airway for delivery, while a more definitive airway is attempted after delivery.

A regional anesthetic may be considered in the obstetric patient with a recognized difficult airway if provisions are made for the unexpected need to induce general anesthesia or secure the airway from complications related to regional anesthesia. The approach to the patient with a recognized difficult airway must consider the urgency of Cesarean section, the skill of the anesthesia provider, and the physical assessment of the patient. Regional techniques may be used as long as the provider recognizes the risk and takes precautions to minimize the likelihood of a high spinal or epidural block and intravascular injection. For example, epidural analgesia may be considered over spinal anesthesia because epidural analgesia may be induced slower with careful monitoring of sensory level. Fiberoptic intubation or other advanced airway techniques may be used in patients with an anticipated difficult airway who have a contraindication to regional anesthesia and therefore require general anesthesia. The nonemergent setting allows time for airway topicalization and securing the airway before induction of general anesthesia in a spontaneously breathing patient.

A failed intubation after induction of general anesthesia, intravascular injection, or cardiac or respiratory arrest requires alternative methods to oxygenate and ventilate the mother. Ventilation with a face mask or laryngeal mask airway (LMA) is therefore used in the setting of an unexpected difficult intubation whereby urgent delivery is necessary due to either a maternal or a fetal emergency (see **Fig. 1**). Further management depends on the experience of the anesthesiologist and the particular patient or obstetric issues unique to that patient, particularly in regards to changing the face mask or LMA to another airway device. Absence of maternal or fetal emergencies affords the opportunity to awaken the patient and perform an awake or regional anesthesia, unless the cause of respiratory distress is related to the regional anesthetic. An unsecured airway in the setting of maternal or fetal emergency requiring urgent Cesarean section demands considerable judgment as to the subsequent management.

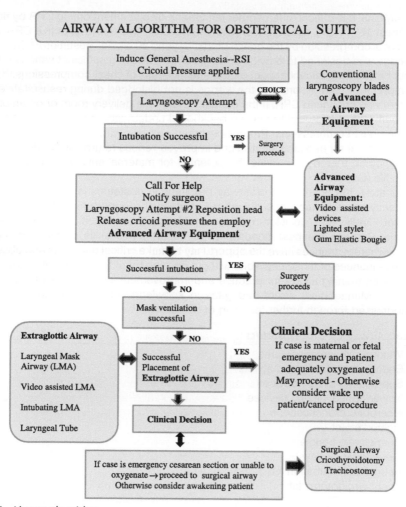

Fig. 1. Airway algorithm.

Each successive intubation attempt should be performed after repositioning the patient and incorporating different techniques or equipment.[18] If ventilation is adequate with an LMA, judgment will have to be made as to whether or not to proceed with the Cesarean section without a protected airway. If there is a higher risk of aspiration (eg, recent large meal), increased risk of desaturation (eg, morbidly obese), or increased risk of subsequent failure to ventilate (traumatized airway with edema), consideration should be made to awaken the mother and perform a regional anesthetic or awake intubation. This approach places the fetus at increased risk of morbidity and mortality and favors management of the mother over the fetus in this difficult clinical dilemma.

Cardiac arrest related to an airway problem is a devastating consequence of the inability to oxygenate and ventilate. Survival of the mother and the fetus depends on performing timely and appropriate resuscitative interventions. Generally the same cardiopulmonary resuscitation (CPR) and advanced cardiac life support algorithms apply to pregnant patients as with nonpregnant patients, with a few modifications. It is critical to remember left uterine displacement during CPR by tilting the patient 15° to 30°, because it is nearly impossible to achieve effective CPR with aorto-caval compression by the gravid uterus beyond 20 weeks' gestation.[19] The Cardiff wedge was designed to provide an angle of 27°, allowing sufficient venous return without having a significant impact on the effectiveness of chest compressions.[20] It is also important to make sure that the wedge is not dislodged during resuscitative efforts involving continued CPR. If the patient is not in the delivery room or on an operating room bed, it is crucial to place a backboard underneath the patient to allow for effective chest compressions. Prompt cesarean delivery (within 5 minutes) provides the best chance for neonatal survival and improves venous return and cardiac output for the mother, thereby improving the potential for maternal survival with advanced cardiac life support.

Fortunately, the occurrence of airway problems in obstetrics is a rare event. The infrequency of exposure does not afford trainees the opportunity to develop the necessary skills and decision-making experience that is critical to successful outcome. Perhaps the best opportunity to impart these skills is with simulation training, whereby trainees have the opportunity to make critical decisions and observe the consequences of those decisions without causing harm to the patient. Multidisciplinary team training allows for practice and improvement in teamwork during crisis situations. Management errors and gaps in knowledge or teaching are identified and addressed through further teaching or discussion.[18]

Difficult Airway Cart for Obstetrics

- Various size laryngoscopes
- Endotracheal tubes and stylets
- Supraglottic airway devices
- Newer optical airway devices
- Fiberoptic bronchoscope
- Lighted stylet
- Gum elastic bougie
- Extraglottic airways
- Retrograde intubation kit
- Cricothyroidotomy kit

Advanced Airway Techniques

Several different airway management techniques must be available in the setting of a difficult airway. The most important factor that predicts success of any airway device is the anesthesiologist's proficiency with that particular tool or approach. Although an algorithm (see **Fig. 1**) was presented in the previous section, there are no widely accepted algorithms for the unanticipated difficult obstetric airway in terms of how to manage such critical cases, although newer algorithms are being developed that incorporate more advanced equipment.

Placement of a supraglottic airway device is used in the setting of an urgent delivery, when both intubation and ventilation are difficult or inadequate to maintain oxygen saturation and a decision has been made regarding use of a nonsurgical versus surgical airway.[6] The LMA (**Fig. 2**) or an extraglottic airway such as a laryngeal tube are both nonsurgical airway options (**Fig. 3**). An LMA is a supraglottic airway device that is easily and quickly inserted to assist in ventilation. The correct size is selected based on the patient's anatomy. Intubation may be performed blindly through the device or with the aid of a fiberoptic bronchoscope. An LMA is easy to use and quickly inserted even by an operator with limited experience.[21] An LMA with an esophageal

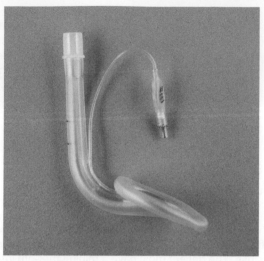

Fig. 2. LMA laryngeal mask airway.

drain can help protect against aspiration and is therefore desirable in the obstetric patient. The LMA Proseal and the LMA Supreme are examples that allow for gastric contents to be aspirated after LMA placement. Some supraglottic airway devices, such as the intubating LMA (**Fig. 4**), allow for passage of a tracheal tube, thus allowing securing of the airway while the LMA is in place (eg, Air-Q and LMA FasTrach).

The recent introduction of modern optical devices has changed the approach to intubation of the difficult airway. These newer devices incorporate a video camera with laryngoscopes, stylets, and LMAs. A large prospective study recently established the validity of incorporating these newer devices into a modified difficult airway algorithm.[22] The use of these devices has changed the way many practitioners approach the difficult airway algorithm. Some practitioners use the video-laryngoscope on their first attempt at intubation, although there are no large trials in obstetric anesthesia to validate this practice (**Fig. 5**).

The video–enhanced LMA (VLMA) has been compared with the other LMA types for ventilation and direct visualization of ETT (endotracheal tube) use through it. Placement of the VLMA in the scenario of "cannot intubate or ventilate" allows for ventilation while providing a view that allows for assessment of the airway. This information then guides clinicians regarding further intubation attempts if structures are not well visualized. Many VLMA provide excellent views of the glottic opening, but placement of the

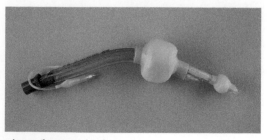

Fig. 3. Extra glottic airway/laryngeal tube.

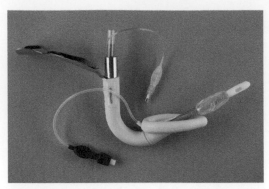

Fig. 4. ILMA intubating LMA.

tracheal tube may be difficult and often requires removal of the tube to ventilate and oxygenate the patient. The VLMA allows for continuous ventilation; however, there are limitations to its use. The patient must have a minimum 3-cm interincisor distance to avoid damage to the teeth.[23] There are other limitations that are important to note, including persistent epiglottic down-folding in extremely tall or obese patients.[23]

The video stylet (VS) is a newer device that is used in conjunction with a laryngoscope. This device allows the practitioner to view the hypopharynx with the laryngoscope, while the VS provides an endoscopic view of the airway simultaneously. The semi-rigid stylet is introduced in the mouth and, once the VS is past the teeth, then the user watches the video monitor and guides the VS through the glottic opening.[24] This device is especially helpful in the unanticipated difficult airway because it allows for direct visualization and avoids traumatic injury to the airway caused by multiple blind intubation attempts.

The video-laryngoscope (VL) has become commonly used in the operating room on a daily basis for routine and potentially difficult intubations. The VL incorporates a video camera at the base of the laryngoscope blade that projects views onto a video screen. The shape of the blade on the VL may vary, but most commonly resembles a Macintosh-type blade with a more acute angle. The ability for several people to view the airway during laryngoscopy makes this a great teaching tool in the operating room with medical students and residents. It is also extremely helpful during a difficult intubation because it allows one to see the anatomy and determine what maneuvers need to be performed to facilitate successful intubation. Although there are no large

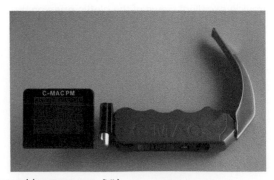

Fig. 5. Video enhanced laryngoscope (VL).

prospective trials comparing this device in the obstetric suite, the VL has demonstrated more successful intubations and earlier recognition of esophageal intubation in the emergency room.[25]

A Combitube (a double lumen tube that is placed in the esophagus) is inserted blindly and often used by nonanesthesia personnel outside of the hospital setting. An inflated cuff occludes the esophagus, while the second lumen allows for ventilation, thereby reducing the likelihood of aspiration of gastric contents into the pulmonary tract. This device is easy to place and does not require direct visualization of the larynx. Aspiration is still a major concern with use of the Combitube and tracheal perforation has been reported.[26] The actual use and success rate using this device during pregnancy is not known. A disadvantage to use of the Combitube is the inability to intubate through this device as is often done with the intubating LMA.

A lighted stylet is another option for a patient with a difficult airway (**Fig. 6**). This is especially useful in the setting of an obstetric patient with a bleeding oropharynx due to thrombocytopenia or multiple intubation attempts, because it does not require visualization of the glottic opening. A lighted stylet relies on the transillumination of the soft tissues of the neck. The light is guided into the trachea after which the preloaded tracheal tube is slid over the stylet into the trachea. Direct visualization of the glottis is not necessary for tracheal tube placement.

The gum elastic bougie (GEB) is another adjunct when the difficult airway is encountered (**Fig. 7**). Another description or name for this device is the tracheal tube introducer or Eschmann stylet. Practitioners become facile with this device through practice and use in a variety of circumstances. The GEB is a solid, but flexible introducer, 60 to 70 cm in length with an angled tip. Smaller studies report differing success rates using the GEB alone or as an adjunct to other supraglottic airways with success rates as low as 20% during difficult intubation.[27] This device may be used with a traditional laryngoscope or VL or passed blindly. The GEB is inserted blindly in the setting of unexpectedly difficult intubation with a grade III or IV view, by use of the tactile sense of the device passing over the ridges of the cartilaginous rings of the trachea. The tracheal tube is then passed over the GEB into the trachea. This device also facilitates passage of a tracheal tube through a supraglottic airway.

Awake fiberoptic intubation is an option in the absence of a maternal or fetal emergency. Fiberoptic bronchoscopes are available as flexible or nonflexible. The rigid fiberoptic Bullard laryngoscope is specifically designed for difficult intubations (**Fig. 8**). The Bullard laryngoscope has been used in an awake obstetric patient.[28] It has a rigid anatomically curved blade with a sheath for the introduction of fiberoptic bundles for illumination, thus making this a rigid and fiberoptic laryngoscope in the

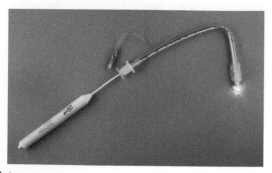

Fig. 6. Lighted stylet.

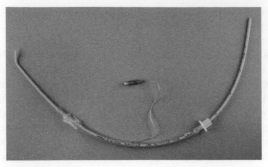

Fig. 7. Gum elastic bougie (GEB).

same apparatus. The Bullard laryngoscope has an eyepiece located on the viewing arm. The handle is connected to a high intensity light source that is transmitted to the distal blade through the fiberoptic bundle. A channel for suction and/or insufflation extends from the body of the scope to the end of the tip. The end nearest the handle has 2 openings: the first is for the Luer-lock connector that is used for suction, insufflation of oxygen, or injection of local anesthetic. The second opening has an attachment for the introducing/intubating stylet, which is thin and curved to the left at approximately 20° near the tip. This brings the end of the stylet into the field of vision and facilitates passage of the tracheal tube into the laryngeal inlet.[29] It allows for visualization of the larynx without the need for aligning the pharyngeal, laryngeal, and oral axes. This device requires less cervical spine manipulation than conventional laryngoscopy and may allow for a more rapid intubation compared with flexible fiberoptic intubation.[30] Patients with blood and secretions that prevent adequate visualization with the flexible fiberoptic laryngoscopy may be intubated with the Bullard laryngoscope because forceful oxygen flow through the insufflation port can effectively clear blood and secretions in the airway. The Bullard laryngoscope has a much larger oxygen insufflation port than the fiberoptic bronchoscope, allowing for more forceful delivery of oxygen.[29] The success with this device, like others, depends on the operator's proficiency and experience.

Flexible fiberoptic intubation is indicated for the expected difficult airway and is also useful for obstetric patients. Fiberoptic bronchoscopes allow for the delivery of supplemental oxygen. A disadvantage to fiberoptic techniques is the expense of the equipment, portability, and the operator's experience and training with use of the

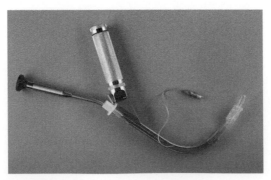

Fig. 8. Bullard™ laryngoscope.

equipment.[6] Successful intubations have been reported in both expected and unexpected difficult obstetric airways based on preoperative evaluation, and for patients with facial abnormalities, facial fractures, goiters, and others. However, placement of a tracheal tube with a fiberoptic bronchoscope in obstetric patients, especially pre-eclamptic patients with laryngeal edema, may result in hypoxia, bleeding from the friable vascular membranes, and trauma to laryngeal structures.[6]

A retrograde intubation technique is another alternative when other less invasive techniques fail. A retrograde technique may be considered in the setting of trauma to the airway from a failed intubation.[31] A guide wire is passed through the crico-thyroid membrane and up into the mouth or nose. This guide wire is then threaded through the suction channel of the fiberoptic scope, which is then advanced along the guide wire to the trachea using fiberoptic visualization.[6]

Surgical interventions for difficult obstetric airways in patients who cannot be ventilated or intubated include tracheal jet ventilation and crico-thyrotomy. Tracheal jet ventilation is a technique whereby a large-bore intravenous catheter is percutaneously placed in the crico-thyroid membrane and highly pressurized oxygen is provided via a jet ventilator. The pressurized oxygen may be delivered from several sources, including directly from the wall outlet. Insufflation of the pressurized oxygen with the jet ventilator achieves inspiration, whereas expiration occurs passively due to the elastic recoil of the lungs.

Crico-thyroidotomy is easier and quicker to perform than a tracheostomy, is associated with fewer complications, and does not require manipulation of the cervical spine. A scalpel is used to make a vertical incision approximately 1 cm in length through the skin and crico-thyroid membrane. The initial incision is further opened by making a 1- to 2-cm horizontal incision. A tracheostomy or tracheal tube is inserted, the cuff is inflated, the tube is secured, and the patient is ventilated.[32]

Emergency situations are unpredictable in the obstetric suite; it is necessary to train all personnel to work together effectively for patient safety. Team training involves all members of the obstetric unit, including obstetricians, anesthesiologists, neonatologists, nurses, residents, and support staff. Communication skills and teamwork are stressed and practiced during emergency scenarios. Regularly scheduled meetings during each shift on the labor suite, attended by all members of the team, allows for all patients to be reviewed and potential problems to be identified prospectively. Multidisciplinary care plans should be developed. It is during these meetings that patients with suspected difficult airways and the team approach are discussed.

Team training reduces the decision to delivery interval for cases of a true emergency.[33] Team training based on crisis resource management alone does not improve safety. Multidisciplinary simulations of obstetric emergencies improve processes of care regardless of whether it occurs in a simulation center or at a local hospital. The most important components of successful training include institutional level incentives to train personnel, multidisciplinary professional training of all staff in the obstetric unit, teamwork training integrated with clinical teaching, and the use of high-fidelity simulation models.[33] Specifically for the anesthesia staff, simulation can be used to practice using the newer airway techniques and to learn the newer airway algorithms. With continued training and vigilance, practitioners can learn to work efficiently and feel more confident when emergencies arise.

SUMMARY

Newer airway techniques have changed the way obstetric airway emergencies are managed. The obstetric anesthesiologist must learn about newer devices and incorporate them in their practice. Because the need for emergent airway management and intubation is mostly unpredictable in the delivery room, anesthesiologists must be organized and prepared at all times. Reviewing, practicing, and adapting emergency airway algorithms as well as becoming proficient in the newest airway devices will help to provide the best outcomes for mother and baby even in the most challenging scenarios.

REFERENCES

1. Deem S, Bishop MJ. Evaluation and management of the difficult airway. Crit Care Clin 1995;11(1):1–26.
2. Quinn AC, Milne D. Failed tracheal intubation in obstetric anaestheisa: 2 yr national case-control study in the UK. Br J Anaesth 2013;110(1):74–80.
3. Mcdonnel NJ, Paech MJ, et al. Difficult and failed intubation in obstetric anaesthesia: an observational study of airway management and complications associated with general anaesthesia for caesarean section. Int J Obstet Anesth 2008; 17:292–7.
4. Rollins M, Lucero J. Overview of anesthetic consideration for Cesarean delivery. Br Med Bull 2012;101:105–25.
5. McClelland SH, Barclay PM. Preoxygenation and apnea in pregnancy: changes during labour and with obstetrical morbidity in a computational simulation. Anaesthesia 2009;64:371–7.
6. Vasdev GM, Harrison BA, et al. Management of the difficult and failed airway in obstetric anesthesia. J Anesth 2008;22:38–48.
7. Edwards N, Middleton PG, et al. Sleep disordered breathing and pregnancy. Thorax 2002;57:555–8.
8. Mhyre J. What's new in obstetric anesthesia in 2003? An update on maternal safety. Anesth Analg 2012;111(6):1480–7.
9. Cheek TG, Baird E. Anesthesia for non-obstetric surgery: maternal and fetal consideration. Clin Obstet Gynecol 2009;52(4):535–45.
10. Munnur U, de Boisblanc B. Airway problems in pregnancy. Crit Care Med 2005; 33(10):s259–68.
11. Samsoon GL, Young JR. Difficult tracheal intubation: a retrospective study. Anaesthesia 1987;42:487–90.
12. Cormack RS, LeHane J. Difficult intubation in obstetrics. Anaesthesia 1984;39: 1105–11.
13. Gonzalez H, Minville V. The importance of neck circumference to intubation difficulties in obese patients. Anesth Analg 2008;166:132–6.
14. American Society of Anesthesiologists Task Force on Obstetric Anesthesia. Practice Guidelines for Obstetric: an updated report by the American Society of Anesthesiologists Task Force on Obstetric Anesthesia. Anesthesiology 2007;106: 843–63.
15. Apfelbaum JL, Hagberg CA, Caplan RA, et al. Practice Guidelines for Management of the Difficult Airway. An updated report by the American Society of Anesthesiologists task force on management of the difficult airway. Anesthesiology 2013;118:251–70.
16. Ezri T, Szmuk P, Evron S, et al. Difficult airway in obstetric anesthesia: a review. Obstet Gynecol Surv 2001;56:631–41.
17. Suresh MS, Wali A. Failed intubation in obstetrics airway management strategies. Anesthesiol Clin North America 1998;16:477–98.

18. Balki M, Cooke ME, Dunington S, et al. Unanticipated difficult airway in obstetric patients. Development of a new algorithm for formative assessment in high-fidelity simulation. Anesthesiology 2012;117:883–97.
19. Campbell TA, Sanson TG. Cardiac arrest and pregnancy. J Emerg Trauma Shock 2009;2:34–42.
20. Peters CW, Layton AJ, Edwards RK. Cardiac arrest during pregnancy. J Clin Anesth 2006;50:27–8.
21. Miller RD. Miller's anesthesia. 6th edition. Philadelphia: Elsevier Churchill Livingstone; 2005. p. 1625–8.
22. Amathieu R, Combes X, et al. An algorithm for difficult airway management, modified for modern optical devices (Airtraq laryngoscope;LMA CTrach) A 2-year prospective validation in patients for elective abdominal, gynecological and thyroid surgery. Anesthesiology 2011;114(1):25–33.
23. Liu EL, Wender R, Goldman AJ. The LMA CTrach™ in patients with difficult airways. Anesthesiology 2009;110:941–3.
24. Biro P, Battig U, Henderson J, et al. First clinical experience of tracheal intubation with the SensaScope™, a novel semi rigid steerable semirigi video stylet. Br J Anaesth 2006;97(2):255–61.
25. Sakles JC, Mosier J, Chiu S, et al. A comparison of the C-MAC video laryngoscope to the Macintosh direct laryngoscope for intubation in the Emergency Department. Ann Emerg Med 2012;60(6):739–48.
26. Klein H, Williamson M, Sue-Ling HM, et al. Esophageal rupture associated with the use of the Combitube. Anesth Analg 1997;85:937–9.
27. Wong DT, Yang JJ, et al. Use of Intubation introducers though a supraglottic airway to facilitate tracheal intubation: a brief review. Can J Anaesth 2012;59: 704–15.
28. Cohn AI, Hart RT, McGraw SR. The Bullard laryngoscope for emergency airway management in a morbidly obese parturient. Anesth Analg 1995;81:872–3.
29. Rionda E, Diaz A, Jimenez A, et al. Intubación orotraqueal con laringoscopio de Bullard. Reporte de 65 cases [Endotracheal intubation with Bullard laryngoscope. A report of 65 cases]. An Med (Mex) 2008;53(3):138–42 [in Spanish].
30. Ghouri AF, Bernstein CA. Use of the Bullard laryngoscope blade in patients with maxillofacial injuries. Anesthesiology 1996;84(2):49.
31. Weksler N, Klein M, Weksler D, et al. Retrograde tracheal intubation: beyond fibreoptic endotracheal intubation. Acta Anaesthesiol Scand 2004;48:412–6.
32. McIntosh SE, Swanson ER, Barton ED. Cricothyrotomy in air medical transport. J Trauma 2008;64(6):1543–7.
33. Mhyre JM, Healy D. The unanticipated difficult airway in obstetrics. Anesth Analg 2011;112(3):648–52.

Improving Communication in the Labor Suite

M. Faith Lukens, MD[a], Regina Y. Fragneto, MD[a,b],*

KEYWORDS

- Communication in obstetrics • Interdisciplinary communication • Team training
- Informed consent • Pain perception • High reliability organization
- Transitions of care • Simulation

KEY POINTS

- Effective communication among providers and between providers and the patient is essential to high-quality obstetric care. Successful communication is the hallmark of a highly reliable obstetric unit.
- Informed consent is an opportunity for shared understanding between patient and provider.
- Providers should be mindful of the terminology they use when communicating with patients regarding painful procedures. The words used by the provider influence the amount of pain experienced by the patient.
- Health care institutions are placing increased emphasis on improving interdisciplinary communication as a means for optimizing patient safety. Team training and simulation on obstetric units are effective tools for improving communication among all providers.

INTRODUCTION

Breakdown in communication is cited as one of the leading problems in patient safety reports. Although inadequate or ineffective communication does not always lead to harm, it may lead to an increase in frustration, cost of care, and delay of treatment. In a retrospective review of one institution's obstetrics and gynecology risk-management files, poor communication was determined to be a potentially preventable contributing factor in almost a third of adverse events.[1] An analysis of obstetric anesthesia closed claims cases also cited poor communication as contributing to neonatal injury or death in over one-third of cases.[2] This review considers not only

Disclosures: Drs Lukens and Fragneto have no disclosures.
[a] Department of Anesthesiology, University of Kentucky College of Medicine, 800 Rose Street, Room N217, Lexington, KY 40536, USA; [b] Obstetric Anesthesia, University of Kentucky College of Medicine, Lexington, KY, USA
* Corresponding author. Department of Anesthesiology, University of Kentucky College of Medicine, 800 Rose Street, Room N217, Lexington, KY 40536.
E-mail address: fragnet@email.uky.edu

Anesthesiology Clin 31 (2013) 545–558
http://dx.doi.org/10.1016/j.anclin.2013.03.003
1932-2275/13/$ – see front matter © 2013 Elsevier Inc. All rights reserved.

strategies to improve communication among multidisciplinary obstetric staff but also ways by which the anesthesiologist may improve communication with patients.

Great advances in patient safety and care by anesthesiologists have been made through improvements in technology and pharmacology; however, there is recent renewed interest in the effect on outcomes of the human factor of communication.[3] A survey of outpatients showed that they placed a value on communication perioperatively, which was undervalued by the anesthesiologist.[4] Obstetric anesthesiologists are in a unique position in that that they are more likely to be remembered for the care they provide than are anesthesiologists in other hospital settings. It is important for the anesthesiologist to consider how he or she communicates with the patient regarding various aspects of care, such as informed consent, pain, or birth plans, as this will have a significant effect on how the woman feels about the birth experience. In fact, women who receive care in patient-centered facilities where they feel they are treated with respect and dignity and are involved in decision making are significantly more likely than women treated in less patient-focused institutions to recommend the facility to their family and friends.[5]

INFORMED CONSENT

Some of the barriers to informed consent should be considered before possible improvements to the process are discussed. While differences in the primary language spoken is an obvious barrier that may exist between provider and patient, less apparent differences also impede the process of informed consent, including different values, beliefs, concerns, cultural backgrounds, and expectations. The patient may expect and request a procedure that the physician is unwilling to perform, such as epidural analgesia to alleviate the pain of labor even if the platelet count is deemed too low. The negative right of the patient to refuse an intervention, such as a cesarean delivery or blood transfusion, must be respected, but a physician does not have to comply with a patient's positive right to request a procedure that may be harmful to her or her fetus.[6,7]

Medicine has moved ethically and legally from the model of physician paternalism whereby the physician made all care decisions that were judged to be in the best interest of the patient, to the current framework of patient autonomy. Within this framework the responsibility of the decision as to what is best for the patient has been shifted to the patient, and the process of informed consent has been developed to provide guidance to the patient when making choices.[6] However, the patient is rarely completely autonomous. She does not possess the medical training or knowledge of the physician, and the physician who is guiding the patient in the decision-making process is not without bias. As the push for increasing autonomy has developed, another change in the process of informed consent has occurred. The standard of information provided in the consent process is no longer the information a reasonable practitioner would be expected to provide, but rather the information a reasonable patient would expect to receive to make a decision regarding a treatment option. There is now a new focus on the patient as the consumer of health care and the physician as the provider.[6]

Some practitioners believe that extreme pain, such as the pain that occurs during labor and delivery, may impede a patient's ability to provide informed consent. Studies looking at recall of information provided to patients in pain show that their ability to mentally and physically consent was not affected by the pain.[6] Some people have even argued that it is not until a woman is in labor that she is fully able to make an informed decision about the pain management technique she wants. In a study that compared women who were retrospectively asked about their decision to undergo epidural analgesia with a similar group of actively laboring women, those who were questioned retrospectively were much more likely to indicate they would refuse an epidural analgesia if the risk of complications was greater than 1 in 10,000. The actively laboring women were far less likely to refuse epidural analgesia, even when presented with the same complication rates and risks as women in the retrospective group. In this study, the laboring women wanted all the risks associated with the epidural disclosed, but the majority did not want the incidence of risks discussed.[8] It is often impractical to disclose every possible risk associated with a procedure, so courts and expert opinion support the discussion of "material risk."[7] This risk relates to the reasonable patient model whereby the type and amount of information disclosed is what most people in similar circumstances would want to know to make an informed decision about the procedure being offered. Risks frequently conveyed in obstetric anesthesia are those that happen with high frequency, are associated with high morbidity, or may have fetal side effects.[7]

Informed consent is a process, and does not end with a signature on a page. The ubiquitous hospital consent forms should be viewed as an impetus for dialogue to occur between patients and physicians. The forms themselves provide very little legal protection if adequate disclosure has not occurred.[6] In the consent process it is important to consider using written information, in addition to verbal disclosure, as this written information helps to improve the patient's understanding and recall of the information disclosed.[9] For example, an informational brochure outlining the risks and benefits of epidural analgesia may be given to women early in labor before they start experiencing severe pain, or even earlier at one of the prenatal visits. An adequate informed consent process increases a patient's satisfaction and participation in her care, whereas a lack of knowledge or feeling of control leads to dissatisfaction with the labor and birth experience.[6,10]

BIRTH PLANS

Woman may present to the Labor and Delivery unit with a written birth plan stating what they desire to have happen during the delivery process. Development of a birth plan is frequently advocated by childbirth educators as a means to improve communication between the patient and health care providers and increase the level of control the patient feels during the birthing process. When developing a birth plan, the patient is asked to consider her options during labor and delivery and to make choices in advance of the birth regarding her desired experience.[11] Unfortunately, a birth plan can have the opposite effect on communication and may cause increased frustration for both patient and providers because of expectations that cannot be met.[12] In a study by Pennell and colleagues,[13] the demographics of women who had birth plans showed that they tended to have a higher level of education (usually college or above), be Caucasian, and be cared for by a certified nurse-midwife. Eighty-nine percent of these women thought that their birth-plan preferences were respected by their nurses and certified nurse-midwives. However, only 66% believed that obstetricians respected their wishes and 68% of anesthesiologists were thought to have respected the patients' preferences.[13] Pain and a sense of lack of control frequently lead to dissatisfaction with the birth experience.[10]

Communication methods to help improve patient understanding and involvement in her care help the woman feel that she has more control over the labor process. Listening to her concerns may reveal opportunities to offer her some control, even if one is unable to meet all her requests.[3] Acknowledgment of her birth plan and being open to discussing it, whether or not the provider agrees with the patient's choices, are a means to reach an understanding between the patient and provider. It provides an opportunity for the patient to express her concerns and desires and for the provider to explain what options are feasible and realistic. With the changing dynamics in the birthing process, patient desires stated in the birth plan may not be able to be met, but on the other hand caregivers should try to facilitate the woman's preferences when possible.[10] Specifically in regard to communication between the patient and anesthesiologist, the most important preference in the birth plan involves the choice about management of labor pain. In one study, more than half of women stated in their birth plan that they did not want pain medications used, but the majority of women requested and received pain medication during their labor. Epidural analgesia was used most commonly, and the women who received an epidural reported a 90% satisfaction rate with their pain management.[13]

PAIN

Patients' perioperative and procedural pain seems to be influenced by the choice of words used by their care providers. The choice of negative or positive wording during the assessment of postoperative pain has a significant effect on the incidence of pain reported, although the choice of words does not necessarily influence the severity of pain when measured on a pain scale.[14] Imaging studies of the brain have demonstrated that pain-evoked activity changes depending on the use of positive or negative words.[14] The choice of words used when questioning a patient about her postoperative experience may influence her perception of whether a sensation she is experiencing is considered pain. This is not to suggest that a patient should not be questioned about her pain level. The provider should consider using phrases with more positive wording, such as "Are you comfortable?" or "How is your recovery going?" versus "What is the severity of your pain?" or "How much are you hurting right now?"

Clinicians will frequently warn patients before potentially painful procedures, such as intravenous or epidural placement, with the intent of preparing patients for the event and alleviating anxiety.[15] However, an increasing body of evidence shows that using words with harsh or negative connotations, such as pain, sting, hurt, or burn, have the opposite undesired effect of increasing patients' perception of pain and their level of anxiety.[11,16] For example, during injection of subcutaneous local anesthetic before neuraxial needle placement, the clinician may use the following phrases to warn the patient there is going to be a "bee sting," "lots of burning" or "a big ouch." These phrases have actually been shown to have a nocebo effect and to heighten the patient's experience of pain or discomfort.[16] Instead the anesthesiologist should consider using a phrase such as "I am going to inject some medicine to numb the area and make you comfortable for the procedure."

IMPROVING PHYSICIAN-PATIENT COMMUNICATION

Recognition that physicians and patients frequently approach their interaction with different agendas is important in understanding communication styles. The patient is often preoccupied with her worries, hopes, and possible consequences of what she is experiencing, whereas the anesthesiologist is interested in gaining the details of the presenting problem. In a study of preanesthetic interviews, more than half of anesthesiologist communication was concerned with getting or giving information while less than 7% was related to emotional aspects of care.[17] Communication between people happens on both a conscious and subconscious level. The main communication styles used by anesthesiologists are direct, logical, and purposeful; that is, conscious communication. Subconscious communication uses both verbal and nonverbal cues to "elicit nonvolitional changes in perception or behavior."[3] For example, during a cesarean delivery with neuraxial anesthesia, a woman may become anxious, stating "I can't breathe." The woman is breathing adequately to be able to converse, but explaining this logic probably would not be as helpful as reassuring her by saying, "It is common after a spinal anesthetic to not be able to feel yourself breathing, but I'm monitoring your oxygen level and it's good."

Women in labor experience an immense array of emotions, and for many the birthing experience is a defining moment in their lives. The labor and delivery unit can be a rewarding but also a demanding and stressful environment for the anesthesiologist. Some strategies recommended by Cyna and colleagues[3] to help facilitate communication include reflective listening, observing, acceptance, utilization, and suggestion. Understanding and using these additional communication strategies help anesthesiologists in their interactions not only with patients but also with other physicians and health care staff. Communication styles that undermine trust and communication with the patient include not paying attention, making untruthful statements, talking down, or disregarding the patient's emotions.[3] Merely telling a patient there is nothing to worry about before undergoing an epidural procedure is unlikely to help, whereas acknowledging the woman's anxiety and then helping her reframe those feelings is beneficial. For example, the anesthesiologist might say, "I know you are worried about the epidural, but I find that most women are surprised by how little they feel once their skin is numb from the local anesthetic." With this statement the anesthesiologist is using suggestion to inform the patient that she too will likely feel very little during epidural placement.

INTERDISCIPLINARY COMMUNICATION IN OBSTETRICS

Over the last 2 decades, evidence has shown that poor interdisciplinary communication contributes significantly to adverse outcomes. Between 1995 and 2005, The Joint Commission (TJC) reported that inadequate communication was the most common root cause of all sentinel events reported to the organization.[18] Specifically for perinatal units, in 2004 TJC issued Sentinel Alert #30, "Preventing infant death and injury during delivery," and found that communication failures played a role in 72% of sentinel events on obstetric units.[19] TJC made improvement in interdisciplinary communication one of its priorities. With health care institutions focusing more attention on the issues of effective staff communication and teamwork, it appears some progress has been made. TJC's most recently published data reported that communication problems were only the third leading root cause identified in sentinel events for the years 2010 to 2012, and during 2011 to 2012, communication failures were found in 60% of sentinel events. For maternal and perinatal sentinel events, however, communication remained the second most common root cause.[20] Information about obstetric anesthesia claims from the American Society of Anesthesiologists Closed Claims Project also indicates that inadequate communication plays an important role in claims associated with serious adverse outcomes. When comparing claims for newborn death or brain damage with or without anesthesia contribution, poor communication occurred more frequently when anesthesia was determined to have played a role in the outcome. Usually this involved inadequate communication between the anesthesiologist and obstetrician regarding the urgency of a cesarean delivery.[2]

BARRIERS TO EFFECTIVE COMMUNICATION AMONG OBSTETRIC TEAM MEMBERS

To develop strategies to improve communication among the many personnel involved in the care of obstetric patients, there must first be an understanding of the barriers that prevent this effective communication. One issue commonly identified is the hierarchical structure that exists on many Labor and Delivery units. The attending obstetrician and/or anesthesiologist is considered the person in charge. Nurses (especially those who are less experienced), technicians, and resident physicians may feel uncomfortable questioning the decisions made by the attending physician. Many factors contribute to these providers' hesitancy, including concerns of being embarrassed or hurting one's reputation if they are wrong, fear of jeopardizing the currently good relationship they may have with the attending physician, fear of retribution or receiving a negative evaluation, and the common human desire to avoid conflict.[21]

Different types of providers might also have been trained to communicate differently. For instance, nurses have generally been taught to be broad and narrative when describing a clinical situation, whereas physicians commonly have learned to be concise, quickly identifying what they believe are the most important issues.[22] These differences in communication styles are likely to interfere with effective communication, especially if the staff is unaware of the differences. Even among physicians of different specialties, communication styles may differ. In one simulation study that investigated the communication strategies of obstetricians and anesthesiologists, significant differences were found. Anesthesiologists were found to use predominantly an advocacy pattern of communication, whereby they would make statements and observations and express opinions; they used an inquiry pattern, eliciting information from others by asking questions, much less frequently. By contrast, obstetricians used a more balanced proportion of advocacy and inquiry patterns. Anesthesiologists advocated patient information and their anesthetic plans in 100% and 93% of the simulation scenarios, respectively, but inquired about patient information and the obstetricians' plans in only 30% and 11% of cases, respectively. The obstetricians advocated patient information and their care plans in 73% of scenarios and asked for patient information and the anesthesiologists' plans in 75% and 59% of cases, respectively.[23]

Effective communication also may be jeopardized by vague communication styles when the health care provider is not explicit about what is needed or who is to complete a task. In debriefing sessions following simulation events, physicians and nurses alike are often surprised to observe how ambiguous they have been when communicating with colleagues. In one study of communication in the operating room, trained observers classified 30% of communication events as communication failures. The types of failures were further categorized as: "occasion" failures, meaning that the timing of the communication was too late to be optimally useful; "content" failures, whereby important information was omitted or inaccurate information was provided; "purpose" failures, whereby either the communication between staff did not result in resolution of the issue or the objective of someone's communication was thought to be inappropriate, such as an attempt at intimidation; and "audience" failures, whereby a key team member was absent during the communication. All types of failures were relatively common, with 45.7% of failures identified as "occasion," 35.7% as "content," 24% as "purpose," and 20.9% as "audience."[24]

Disruptive behavior by health care professionals is another serious contributing factor to ineffective interdisciplinary communication. Such behavior has been defined by the American Medical Association as "a style of interaction…that interferes with patient care…and tends to cause distress among other staff and affect overall morale within the work environment, undermining productivity and possibly leading to high staff turnover or even resulting in ineffective or substandard care."[25] Other staff are often intimidated by the disruptive professional, resulting in a reluctance to communicate patient concerns or suggestions for patient care, which ultimately compromises patient safety. Although it has been estimated that only 3% to 5% of health care professionals demonstrate disruptive behavior,[26] a survey of obstetric units in the Pacific Northwest suggests that they have a disproportionately negative effect on their work environments. In this survey, 61% of responding units indicated disruptive behavior by a health care professional had occurred, and on 75% of those units the behavior occurred at least monthly. Team members from all disciplines, including physicians, nurses, nurse-midwives, and nurse-anesthetists, were identified as offenders. Especially concerning was the perception of those surveyed that hospital administration was not usually effective in addressing the disruptive behavior.[27] It does appear, however, that professional organizations are paying more attention to this problem. The American College of Obstetricians and Gynecologists has published a Committee Opinion addressing the issue.[28]

STRATEGIES TO IMPROVE INTERDISCIPLINARY COMMUNICATION IN OBSTETRICS

Programs and ideas from other industries focused on improving communication and team behavior have been adapted to health care in an attempt to improve patient safety. One of these ideas is the concept of high-reliability organizations, such as aviation, nuclear power, and the technical aspects of banking, which operate highly complex systems without mistakes for long periods of time.[29] Similar to the characteristics of these other highly reliable industries, a perinatal unit is considered highly reliable if: (1) safety is the predominant theme of the unit's culture and is the duty of all staff; (2) patient safety is considered a team responsibility; (3) respectful communication is highly valued; and (4) obstetric emergencies are rehearsed and unexpected occurrences are anticipated.[30] The following conditions are necessary to achieve a highly reliable obstetric unit (**Box 1**): professional behavior, common goals, clear communication, lack of hierarchy, multidisciplinary transparency in decision making, and teamwork. Effective communication is certainly one of the most important characteristics of a high-reliability organization. Communication among health care providers must be clear, respectful, direct, and explicit (**Box 2**). When a provider has a concern about a patient care plan, the provider must state the concerns to the other providers, request a rationale for the plan, and be willing to listen to other providers' reasons for their decisions.[31]

Several strategies have been used throughout the United States and Europe to improve communication and teamwork on Labor and Delivery units, including crisis (or crew) resource management (CRM), other team-training programs, and simulation. Staff participation in at least 2 of these programs will likely lead to a great improvement in interdisciplinary communication and team behavior on the obstetric unit.

Box 1
Necessary conditions for a highly reliable perinatal unit

- Professional behavior
- Common goals
- Effective communication
- Lack of hierarchy
- Multidisciplinary transparency in decision making
- Teamwork

Box 2
Communication characteristics within a highly reliable perinatal unit

- Clear
- Respectful
- Direct
- Explicit

TRANSITIONS OF CARE

Transitions of care are a frequent occurrence on the Labor and Delivery unit. Shift change is no longer just a common event between nursing staff, but increasingly is happening among residents and faculty as work patterns have changed. The following is used as a definition of clinical handovers: "the transfer of information and professional responsibility and accountability between individuals and teams, within the overall system of care."[32] If there is a breakdown in communication with missing or inaccurate information or a delay in acceptance of responsibility for a patient's care, mistakes or patient harm may occur. Patient outcomes have been linked to the quality of clinical handovers.[32,33] Barriers to effective clinical handovers include incomplete or inaccurate information, distractions occurring during transfer, absence of all team members, absent or incomplete performance of clinical tasks, and/or lack of standardization.[33]

With the increasing scrutiny of transitions of care as an error-prone time and the increasing number of handovers being performed because of limitations on work hours, the literature on this subject is mounting. The multidisciplinary structure of the Labor and Delivery unit makes it particularly important that information is shared effectively not only between anesthesiologists but also among obstetricians, nurses, neonatologists, and midwives. Researchers have looked outside of health care to high-fidelity enterprises such as the aviation industry as role models for the standardization of processes and error reduction.[34] Checklists have been advocated as a method to standardize handovers and work processes to reduce variance in work and omission of information. Components of a good clinical handover include: a systematic approach; protected time; use of both verbal and written information; not performing other tasks simultaneously; and allowing time for questions and answers.[33,35]

Transfer of responsibility of care for the patient is regularly an assumed part of the handover. However, for many physicians there may be an ambiguous time when they still feel responsibility toward a patient even after giving a report to another team member. For some clinicians it is only when they have physically left the hospital that they feel responsibility is transferred; for others it is when they have shared all relevant information regarding a patient, even if this involves calling the hospital to communicate information they had previously forgotten to include in the handover.[36] Ambiguity of responsibility results in problems, especially in cases of escalation in patient care, such as an emergency cesarean delivery. When and whom to notify is not always clear, which may lead to delays and possible patient harm.[32] This possibility for ambiguity emphasizes the importance during clinical handovers of the members of the same specialty understanding the transfer of responsibility. Also, a multidisciplinary means for all team members involved in that patient's care to know that responsibility has been transferred is critical, so that wasted time and delay of care caused by contacting the wrong person is avoided.

Establishment of well-structured, consistently executed handovers between staff requires support and advocacy from administration and involvement of front-line clinical personnel in all phases of both the development and implementation of the process. Although transitions of care are frequently error-prone times, it is important to be aware that structured interdisciplinary handovers actually serve as a time when potential problems are recognized.[37] The unrecognized slow deterioration of clinical status, a phenomenon known as "inattentional blindness," may be recognized by the new personnel assuming responsibility during a transition of care.[38] When the process for improving transitions of care on the obstetrics unit is developed, the informational or technical component of the handover, as well as the human factors or nontechnical component, need to be established and monitored. The technical component of a clinical handover refers to the informational checklists used in the transfer, such as SBAR (Situation-Background-Assessment-Recommendations), whereas the human-factors aspect of a handover refers to the communication quality, teamwork, leadership, situational awareness, and task-management components of the handover.[39]

CRISIS RESOURCE MANAGEMENT

CRM was first used in the aviation industry, and anesthesiologists were the first to adapt this program to train health care providers in the principles of effective teamwork and communication for use in urgent, stressful clinical situations.[40] As CRM training has become more widely accepted in health care, it has become clear that the skills learned through this program are useful in all aspects of patient care. The philosophy behind CRM is that the behaviors necessary for a team to work effectively are identifiable and teachable. In addition, team members do not innately possess these behaviors. To practice the identified behaviors reliably and regularly, members of the health care team must receive specific training and reinforcement in the principles of CRM.[41] Effective communication is the central tenet of CRM and is necessary to achieve the other important components of the CRM concept, including task management, working as a team, situation awareness, and decision making (**Fig. 1**). CRM has been taught in a variety of ways. Seminar-based courses that include didactics and team-building exercises have been used.[41] Within the anesthesiology and obstetrics communities, it is more common to incorporate simulation along with the didactics and group exercises of CRM training. Research has demonstrated the effectiveness of CRM in obstetrics. At one institution, 4 teams participated in a postpartum hemorrhage simulation. Only 2 of these teams then underwent CRM training. The hemorrhage simulation was later repeated for all groups. Improvement in team communication during the second simulation was found only for those teams that had participated in the CRM training. Specifically, team members from these groups more frequently used directed communication whereby a task assignment was directed to a specific person, with that person acknowledging both the request and completion of the task.[42]

Other team-training programs are also available for health care providers. The United States Agency for Healthcare Research and Quality has developed the TeamSTEPPS program[43] that has been used by many health care institutions. In addition, some Labor and Delivery units have used simulation exercises, both on the unit itself and at simulation centers, without incorporating a formal team-training program, such as CRM.

LANGUAGE PATTERNS TO IMPROVE INTERDISCIPLINARY COMMUNICATION

As already discussed, barriers to effective communication include the use of vague communication styles, leading to communication failures and the hesitancy of some

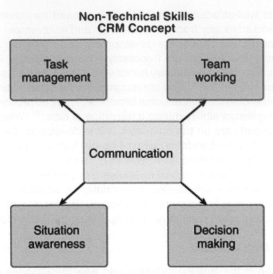

Non-Technical Skills
CRM Concept

Task management

Team working

Communication

Situation awareness

Decision making

Fig. 1. Key components of crisis resource management (CRM), with communication as the core principle. (*From* Rall M, Gaba DM, Howard SK, et al. Human performance and patient safety. In: Miller RD, editor. Miller's anesthesia. 7th edition. Philadelphia: Churchill Livingstone; 2010. p. 106, Figs. 6–7; with permission.)

team members to speak up because of a hierarchical structure. Strategies to teach staff language patterns that resolve these problems and improve communication are available. Most health care providers are familiar with the SBAR formula for providing effective patient handovers. Use of this or another standardized form of communication should be encouraged for all patient-care communications on the Labor and Delivery unit, not just handovers. Such standardized language would lead to clearer, more precise communication. Failures of content and purpose would especially be minimized by all staff adopting such a communication style.

Overcoming the hesitancy of some team members to speak up may not be easy to overcome. CRM training and the goal of becoming a highly reliable perinatal unit are both meant to flatten the hierarchy that seems almost ubiquitous in health care. Practical strategies are necessary to realize assertive communication by all health care personnel. Successful techniques that use the teaching of specific language patterns as part of a simulation debriefing session have been reported. In one study, anesthesiology residents participated in an obstetric emergency simulation during which opportunities arose to challenge an attending physician or nurse. During the debriefing session, the simulation instructors engaged the residents in a discussion of why they were reluctant to challenge another health care provider, and emphasized their obligation to speak up. The concept of the 2-challenge rule (again adopted from the aviation industry) was introduced, whereby any team member has the obligation to speak up and question a patient-care plan if they feel something is wrong. If no response occurs after making 2 challenges to the other provider, the team member is expected to seek help from someone else in resolving the situation. Important in the debriefing session, however, was further education regarding the use of language that pairs advocacy and inquiry. The resident was instructed, when using the 2-challenge rule, to state his opinion (advocacy) but then ask in a genuinely curious manner what the other provider's thoughts are regarding the situation (inquiry). Research in organizational behavior has shown that such an approach is likely to minimize the other provider's defensiveness when challenged, and increase his receptiveness to the resident's concern. After undergoing the simulation debriefing, the residents participated in a different obstetric emergency simulation during which the opportunity to challenge another health care provider again occurred. The investigators found a marked improvement in the quality of the residents' challenges as a result of using the advocacy-inquiry language they had been taught.[21]

Another recent study involved the use of invitational medical rhetoric (IMR) training to improve communication and teamwork among obstetric team members. Obstetricians and anesthesiologists first participated in an obstetric high-fidelity simulation session, followed by an educational session that included a discussion of common rhetoric and speaking styles that lead to alienation and silencing of team members, as well as an introduction to IMR. With IMR, health care providers are taught language choices that promote effective interdisciplinary communication and team behaviors. A subsequent simulation session was conducted following the teaching of IMR. Scoring of the physicians' communication during this session found that after instruction in IMR, language promoting interdependence and integration of team members increased, whereas language suggesting an independent approach to patient management decreased.[44]

INTERDISCIPLINARY COMMUNICATION DURING OBSTETRIC EMERGENCIES

Effective communication among obstetric team members is essential to optimize patient outcomes during obstetric emergencies. Many institutions have implemented programs to improve communication and teamwork among obstetric care providers during these emergencies. In most published reports high fidelity simulation sessions and team training that includes formal, didactic teaching about communication and team behavior principles have been used.[45–50] The equipment and personnel costs for this training is expensive, so organizations will understandably be reluctant to adopt such programs without clear evidence that they result in improved patient safety and outcomes.

Until recently, most data that were available to evaluate the effectiveness of these team-training exercises in health care were assessments or surveys completed by the participants and observers indicating improved interdisciplinary communication and teamwork. Some recent studies in obstetrics, however, have reported on objective data supporting the usefulness of team-training programs for improving performance during emergencies. In the Netherlands, obstetric teams were assigned to an intervention or control group, with the intervention group participating in team training at a simulation center. Several months later, in situ simulations of obstetric emergencies were conducted for all teams. Those from the intervention group not only scored higher than the control group on a clinical teamwork scale, indicating improved communication and decision making, but they were also significantly more likely to perform a perimortem cesarean delivery within 5 minutes in an amniotic fluid embolism scenario (83% vs 46%).[48] In the United States a large Labor and Delivery unit (>9000 deliveries/year) implemented a CRM and simulation training program in which nearly 75% of their nurses, obstetricians, midwives, and anesthesia providers participated. The adverse outcomes index before and after initiating the team-training program were compared. A significant decrease in the index occurred in the period following implementation of the training.[49] A systematic review of 8 studies investigating simulation and multidisciplinary team training for obstetric emergencies showed improvement in communication and team performance. Although only 1 of the studies reported on patient outcomes, it found decreases in the rates of low Apgar scores and neonatal hypoxic-ischemic encephalopathy after the implementation of simulation-based team training. Many hospitals, however, may not have the capability to send most of their staff to a simulation center to train for obstetric emergencies. Perhaps the conclusion from this systematic review that simulation training at a simulation center was not superior to in situ simulation performed on one's own Labor and Delivery unit was one of its most important findings.[50]

SUMMARY

Improved communication is a mantra that has been embraced worldwide by many stakeholders within health care systems; it certainly is a goal for which all care providers of pregnant women must strive. The obstetric anesthesiologist, in particular, is in an influential position to advocate for and effect change that leads to improved communication on the Labor and Delivery unit. Anesthesiologists are integral to both the safety and satisfaction of patients receiving care on the obstetrics unit. For change to occur there must first be an understanding of the barriers to effective communication, whether it is structural hierarchy, differences in communication styles, or disorganized information transfers. With this knowledge, the anesthesiologist evaluates the current methods of communication and takes steps to become a more effective communicator with both patients and other care providers. A personal ambition to improve communication is often a catalyst to becoming involved in instituting systems-based changes aimed at increasing effective multidisciplinary communication. Tools such as team training, CRM, standardization of communication styles, and teaching of IMR are all available to improve communication on the Labor and Delivery unit.

REFERENCES

1. White AA, Pichert JW, Bledsoe SH, et al. Cause and effect analysis of closed claims in obstetrics and gynecology. Obstet Gynecol 2005;105:1031–8.
2. Davies JM, Posner KL, Lee LA, et al. Liability associated with obstetric anesthesia: a closed claims analysis. Anesthesiology 2009;110:131–9.
3. Cyna AM, Andrew MI, Tan SG. Communication skills for the anaesthetist. Anaesthesia 2009;64:658–65.
4. Fung D, Cohen M. What do outpatients value most in their anesthesia care? Can J Anaesth 2001;48:12–9.
5. Harriott EM, Williams TV, Peterson MR. Childbearing in U.S. military hospitals: dimensions of care affecting women's perceptions of quality and satisfaction. Birth 2005;32:4–10.
6. Hoehner PJ. Ethical aspects of informed consent in obstetric anesthesia—new challenges and solutions. J Clin Anesth 2003;15:587–600.
7. Broaddus BM, Chandrasekhar S. Informed consent in obstetric anesthesia. Anesth Analg 2011;112:912–5.
8. Jackson A, Henry R, Avery N, et al. Informed consent for labour epidurals: what labouring women want to know. Can J Anaesth 2000;47:1068–73.
9. Middle JV, Wee MY. Informed consent for epidural analgesia in labour: a survey of UK practice. Anaesthesia 2009;64:161–4.
10. Fowles ER. Labor concerns of women two months after delivery. Birth 1998;25:235–40.
11. Simpson KR, James DC, Knox GE. Nurse-physician communication during labor and birth: implications for patient safety. J Obstet Gynecol Neonatal Nurs 2006;35:547–56.

12. Lothian J. Birth plans: the good, the bad, and the future. J Obstet Gynecol Neonatal Nurs 2006;35:295–303.
13. Pennell A, Salo-Coombs V, Herring A, et al. Anesthesia and analgesia-related preferences and outcomes of women who have birth plans. J Midwifery Womens Health 2011;56:376–81.
14. Chooi CS, Nerlekar R, Raju A, et al. The effects of positive or negative words when assessing postoperative pain. Anaesth Intensive Care 2011;39:101–6.
15. Dutt-Gupta J, Bown T, Cyna AM. Effect of communication on pain during intravenous cannulation: a randomized controlled trial. Br J Anaesth 2007;99:871–5.
16. Varelmann D, Pancaro C, Cappiello EC, et al. Nocebo-induced hyperalgesia during local anesthetic injection. Anesth Analg 2010;110:868–70.
17. Hool A, Smith AF. Communication between anaesthesiologists and patients: how are we doing it now and how can we improve? Curr Opin Anaesthesiol 2009;22:431–5.
18. O'Byrne WT 3rd, Weavind L, Selby J. The science and economics of improving clinical communication. Anesthesiol Clin 2008;26:729–44.
19. The Joint Commission. Preventing infant death and injury during delivery. Sentinel Event Alert 2004;21:30.
20. The Joint Commission. Sentinel event data. Available at: http://www.joint commission.org/sentinel_event.aspx. Accessed February 23, 2013.
21. Pian-Smith MC, Simon R, Minehart RD, et al. Teaching residents the two-challenge rule: a simulation-based approach to improve education and patient safety. Simul Healthc 2009;4:84–91.
22. Leonard M, Graham S, Bonacum D. The human factor: the critical importance of effective teamwork and communication in providing safe care. Qual Saf Health Care 2004;13(Suppl 1):i85–90.
23. Minehart RD, Pian-Smith MC, Walzer TB, et al. Speaking across the drapes: communication strategies of anesthesiologists and obstetricians during a simulated maternal crisis. Simul Healthc 2012;7:166–70.
24. Lingard L, Espin S, Whyte S, et al. Communication failures in the operating room: an observational classification of recurrent types and effects. Qual Saf Health Care 2004;13:330–4.
25. American Medical Association. Physicians with disruptive behavior. In: Code of medical ethics: current opinions and annotations. 2010-11 edition. Chicago: AMA; 2010. p. 326–8.
26. Leape LL, Fromson JA. Problem doctors: is there a system-level solution? Ann Intern Med 2006;17(144):107–15.
27. Veltman LL. Disruptive behavior in obstetrics: a hidden threat to patient safety. Am J Obstet Gynecol 2007;196:587.e1–4 [discussion: 587.e4–5].
28. ACOG Committee Opinion No. 508: disruptive behavior. Obstet Gynecol 2011; 118:970–2.
29. Knox GE, Simpson KR, Garite TJ. High reliability perinatal units: an approach to the prevention of patient injury and medical malpractice claims. J Health Risk Manag 1999;19:24–32.
30. Knox GE, Simpson KR. Perinatal high reliability. Am J Obstet Gynecol 2011;204: 373–7.
31. Lyndon A, Zlatnik MG, Wachter RM. Effective physician-nurse communication: a patient safety essential for labor and delivery. Am J Obstet Gynecol 2011;205: 91–6.
32. Jeffcott SA, Evans SM, Cameron PA, et al. Improving measurement in clinical handover. Qual Saf Health Care 2009;18:272–7.

33. Segall N, Bonifacio AS, Schroeder RA, et al, Patient Safety Center of Inquiry. Can we make postoperative patient handovers safer? A systematic review of the literature. Anesth Analg 2012;115:102–15.

34. Haynes AB, Weiser TG, Berry WR, et al, Safe Surgery Saves Lives Study Group. Changes in safety attitude and relationship to decreased postoperative morbidity and mortality following implementation of a checklist-based surgical safety intervention. BMJ Qual Saf 2011;20:102–7.

35. Jorm CM, White S, Kaneen T. Clinical handover: critical communications. Med J Aust 2009;190(Suppl 11):S108–9.

36. Chin GS, Warren N, Kornman L, et al. Transferring responsibility and accountability in maternity care: clinicians defining their boundaries of practice in relation to clinical handover. BMJ Open 2012;4:2.

37. Manser T, Foster S, Gisin S, et al. Assessing the quality of patient handoffs at care transitions. Qual Saf Health Care 2010;19:e44.

38. Edozien LC. Structured multidisciplinary intershift handover (SMITH): a tool for promoting safer intrapartum care. J Obstet Gynaecol 2011;31:683–6.

39. Pezzolesi C, Manser T, Schifano F, et al. Human factors in clinical handover: development and testing of a 'handover performance tool' for doctors' shift handovers. Int J Qual Health Care 2013;25:58–65.

40. Howard SK, Gaba DM, Fish KJ, et al. Anesthesia crisis resource management training: teaching anesthesiologists to handle critical incidents. Aviat Space Environ Med 1992;63:763–70.

41. Morey JC, Simon R, Jay GD, et al. Error reduction and performance improvement in the emergency department through formal teamwork training: evaluation results of the MedTeams project. Health Serv Res 2002;37:1553–81.

42. Siassakos D, Draycott T, Montague I, et al. Content analysis of team communication in an obstetric emergency scenario. J Obstet Gynaecol 2009;29:499–503.

43. United States Department of Health and Human Services. Agency for Healthcare Research and Quality. TeamSTEPPS: national implementation. Available at: http://teamstepps.ahrq.gov. Accessed February 24, 2013.

44. Kirschbaum KA, Rask JP, Brennan M, et al. Improved climate, culture, and communication through multidisciplinary training and instruction. Am J Obstet Gynecol 2012;207:200.e1–7.

45. Daniel LT, Simpson EK. Integrating team training strategies into obstetrical emergency simulation training. J Healthc Qual 2009;31:38–42.

46. Clark EA, Fisher J, Arafeh J, et al. Team training/simulation. Clin Obstet Gynecol 2010;53:265–77.

47. Robertson B, Schumacher L, Gosman G, et al. Simulation-based crisis team training for multidisciplinary obstetric providers. Simul Healthc 2009;4:77–83.

48. Fransen AF, van de Ven J, Merién AE, et al. Effect of obstetric team training on team performance and medical technical skills: a randomised controlled trial. BJOG 2012;119:1387–93.

49. Phipps MG, Lindquist DG, McConaughey, et al. Outcomes from a labor and delivery team training program with simulation component. Am J Obstet Gynecol 2012;206:3–9.

50. Merién AE, van de Ven J, Mol BW, et al. Multidisciplinary team training in a simulation setting for acute obstetric emergencies: a systematic review. Obstet Gynecol 2010;115:1021–31.

Epidural Analgesia and Maternal Fever: Real or Fiction?

Abha A. Shah, MD*, Grace H. Shih, MD

KEYWORDS

- Labor • Obstetric anesthesia • Epidural fever • Epidural analgesia • Maternal fever
- Neonatal sepsis • Temperature regulation • Epidural inflammation

KEY POINTS

- The evidence suggests that there is a relationship between epidural analgesia and maternal fever during labor; however, it is not a cause-and-effect relationship.
- Most studies have shown that epidural fevers during labor are unlikely to have an infectious cause. They may be the result of inflammation and/or altered thermoregulation.
- In the absence of maternal fever, there is no proven association between epidural analgesia and neonatal sepsis evaluation.

INTRODUCTION

Maternal intrapartum fever is defined as an increase of core body temperature to greater than 37.5 to 38°C and has been associated with up to one-third of all deliveries. There is a wide range of causes of maternal fever, which can be divided into infectious and noninfectious causes. Although infection is still the most common etiology, studies have suggested an association between epidural analgesia in labor and maternal fevers. Early recognition of maternal fever is important, because fever is associated with maternal and neonatal consequences. This article focuses on the causes of maternal fever with a detailed discussion of epidural-associated fever.

NORMAL MATERNAL TEMPERATURE MEASUREMENTS

Maternal temperature is measured routinely during labor to identify fever in a timely fashion. There have been several studies of temperature variations for normal

Funding Sources: Nil.
Conflict of Interest: Nil.
Department of Anesthesiology, University of Kansas Medical Center, 3901 Rainbow Boulevard, Kansas City, KS 66160, USA
* Corresponding author.
E-mail address: ashah3@kumc.edu

full-term parturients. Acker and colleagues[1] studied admission temperatures in the 1980s for parturients and found that temperatures ranged from 34.6 to 37.6°C.

Bartholomew and colleagues[2] found that labor alone did not significantly increase normal body temperature and described a mean temperature of 37.0°C during labor. Their study was a retrospective chart review of 147 patients, and temperatures were measured sublingually. They found no difference in the maximum temperatures of patients who did and did not receive prophylactic antibiotics during labor.

Schouten and colleagues[3] performed a larger prospective study including more than 3000 patients. Temperatures were measured rectally every 2 to 3 hours, and the average temperature at the beginning of labor was 37.1°C for all patients. Temperatures remained stable for patients in the normal labor group, although the definition of normal labor was narrow and only included 27% of the total patients studied. The normal labor group included parturients at greater than 37 weeks' gestation with a spontaneous onset of labor, ruptured membranes less than 18 hours, clear amniotic fluid, and normal labor progression without augmentation resulting in spontaneous delivery of a healthy infant. All other patients, including patients given antibiotics or epidural analgesia, were placed in the abnormal labor group. Patients in the abnormal labor group, which represented most patients, showed a small increase in temperature to 37.4°C after 22 hours.

Froelich and colleagues[4] found a significant linear trend of temperature increase over time in 81 laboring women without signs of infection. Temperatures were measured orally every hour. The overall trend in temperature increase was small, with an average of 0.2°C over 10 hours of labor.

Banerjee and colleagues[5] studied the best noninvasive monitor to reflect intrauterine temperature. They enrolled 18 patients and measured simultaneous uterine, tympanic, and skin surface temperatures every 10 seconds and oral temperatures every hour throughout labor. Oral temperature measurements had the best correlation with uterine temperature. On average, oral temperature underestimated intrauterine temperature by 0.8°C. Oral temperatures of greater than 37.2°C detected an intrauterine temperature greater than 38°C with a sensitivity of 81% and a specificity of 96%. Oral temperatures have been thought to be unreliable in the past because of variability with consumption of hot and cold drinks or ice chips. Banerjee and colleagues[5] accounted for this by ensuring that the oral thermometer was in place for at least 2 minutes and by not allowing cold water, ice chips, or hot drinks for at least 15 minutes before the measurement. They thought that, using this technique, oral temperature gave a reasonable estimate of intrauterine temperature and potential thermal stress to the fetus.

Summarizing this literature, most patients seem to have a linear increase in temperature during labor. Normal maternal temperatures during labor range from 36.4 to 37.6°C. Most of the literature defines maternal fever as oral maternal temperatures greater than 38°C. Oral temperature measurements correlate well with intrauterine temperatures when obtained using good technique. The intrauterine environment has slightly higher temperatures than those measured orally.

LABOR EPIDURAL ANALGESIA FEVER

Many recent studies have shown that, in laboring women, epidural analgesia has been associated with a gradual increase in maternal temperature. A variety of study designs have been used to determine the association between epidural analgesia and maternal fever. Depending on the type of study, selection bias may be a factor in the outcome of the trial. Women who choose epidural analgesia may be at risk for increase in temperature from other causes such as dysfunctional labor.

Uncontrolled Studies

Fusi and colleagues[6] were some of the first investigators to study maternal temperature changes associated with epidural analgesia. They specifically studied temperature increase after epidural catheter placement. They showed that vaginal temperature began to increase 1 hour after epidural insertion at a rate of approximately 1°C over 7 hours. The temperatures were similar in the two groups before epidural placement and temperatures remained constant in the nonepidural group. The study group was small, with 18 women in the epidural group and 15 women in the intramuscular meperidine group. They showed good correlation between oral and vaginal temperatures.

Herbst and colleagues[7] conducted a larger study of 3109 patients in both a retrospective case-control study and matched-pair study, and 83% of patients with epidural analgesia developed fever versus 53% of controls. Sixty-two percent of the patients with fever had an epidural catheter, whereas 21% of afebrile patients had one. In the case-control study, nulliparity and long duration of labor were associated with increased temperatures. In the matched-pair study, ruptured membranes greater than 24 hours, temperature in the upper normal range on arrival, and a long interval from arrival to established labor were independent risk factors for fever. Both studies showed that epidural analgesia was independently associated with maternal fever.

Lieberman and colleagues[8] studied 1657 patients in a secondary analysis of women who were randomized to active management of labor. Of the patients with epidural analgesia, 14.5% developed fever versus 1% of controls. With logistic regression analysis, maternal fever was associated with epidural use.

Other studies also have shown an association between epidural analgesia and maternal fever. Gonen and colleagues[9] performed an observational study of 1004 patients, 40% of whom received epidural analgesia. Twelve percent of the patients who received epidural analgesia developed a fever versus 0.2% in patients without. Ninety-eight percent of maternal fevers occurred in patients with epidural analgesia. With logistic regression analysis, the duration of epidural analgesia was the only thing to be associated with maternal fever occurrence.

Yancey and colleagues[10] performed a retrospective analysis of before the immediate availability of epidural analgesia and after in a tertiary care medical center of more than 1000 patients. Incidence of epidural analgesia was 1% before and only available for patients deemed to have a medical indication. After epidural analgesia became available on request, the incidence of labor epidural analgesia increased to 83%. The increased use of epidural analgesia resulted in a 20-fold increase in the incidence of intrapartum fever of at least 38.0°C (100.4°F).

Macaulay and colleagues[11] prospectively studied fetal skin, maternal uterine wall, and maternal oral cavity temperatures. Patients received epidural analgesia on request. Patients with epidural analgesia were more likely to have uterine temperatures greater than 37.5°C. Fetal temperature correlated with duration of epidural analgesia. Oral temperatures underestimated fetal temperatures in 95% of cases.

Controlled Studies

Several controlled trials have also studied the association between epidural use and intrapartum fever. Philip and colleagues[12] analyzed 715 women randomized to epidural versus intravenous analgesia and found a significant increase in fever associated with epidural (15%) versus intravenous analgesia (4%). When stratified according to parity, fever was more common in nulliparous women receiving epidural analgesia but not in multiparous women compared with controls. Prolonged labor also was independently associated with maternal fever.

As in the study by Lieberman and colleagues,[8] this was a secondary analysis of another study. Unlike the study by Lieberman and colleagues,[8] this study randomized patients to either epidural analgesia or intravenous medications, whereas the study by Lieberman and colleagues[8] allowed patients to self-select the method of analgesia. By allowing patients to self-select their analgesia, selection bias may have had an effect on the results. Patients who request epidural analgesia are more likely to have longer, dysfunctional, painful labors or require induction of labor. These factors alone increase the incidence of maternal fever.[13]

Camann and colleagues[14] prospectively studied 53 women in active labor. No differences in temperatures were noted during the first 4 hours. Patients with epidural analgesia had greater tympanic membrane temperatures after 5 hours of epidural analgesia than those who received parenteral opioids.

Other studies with different end points have also noted an association between epidural analgesia and maternal fever.

Dashe and colleagues[15] prospectively studied 149 consecutive patients, specifically examining placental disorders. Fifty-four percent of patients received epidural analgesia, and 46% of patients who developed fever had epidural analgesia versus 26% who did not.

De Orange and colleagues[16] prospectively randomized 70 women to either combined spinal-epidural analgesia (CSE) or nonpharmacologic methods of pain control. There was a significant increase in median maternal temperature as early as 1 hour after CSE analgesia, which disappeared after 6 hours of labor. This increase was not observed in the nonpharmacologic group. Fifteen percent of the CSE group had a fever, compared with no patients in the nonpharmacologic group.

Sharma and colleagues[17] performed a randomized trial of 459 women to determine whether there was a difference in cesarean section rates between epidural analgesia and intravenous meperidine use for labor analgesia. They also analyzed several other variables, including maternal fever (defined as temperature $>38°C$). Although they did not find a difference in cesarean section rate, they did note a statistically significant higher incidence of maternal fever (33% vs 7%) in the epidural analgesia group.

Mantha and colleagues[18] compared maternal temperatures in women randomized to intermittent labor epidural analgesia (ILEA) versus continuous labor epidural analgesia (CLEA). The incidence of fever ($>38°C$) in the ILEA group was significantly lower at 4 hours (2/42 vs 10/44). No significant differences were detected at other time points.

Combination Studies

Vinson and colleagues[19] performed a retrospective chart review of women in labor, a prospective cohort study of women in labor, and a case-control study of newborns with fever. Maximum maternal temperature greater than or equal to 38.0°C was 15% in patients who received epidural analgesia in the retrospective group and 7% in the prospective group. The duration of epidural analgesia correlated with maximum maternal temperature with an increase in temperature of 0.07°C per hour of exposure to epidural analgesia.

MECHANISM OF INCREASED MATERNAL TEMPERATURE

In general, fever is most likely a resetting of the hypothalamic thermoregulatory center in response to pyrogens such as infection, inflammation, injury, or an antigenic challenge. The mechanism of the increased maternal temperatures during labor, especially in conjunction with epidural analgesia, remains controversial. Several theories have been suggested, including (1) infection, (2) alteration in thermoregulation, and (3) inflammation.

Infection

Infection is the most common cause of increased temperature or maternal fever in labor. One of the most concerning infections during labor is chorioamnionitis because of its association with neonatal sepsis. Chorioamnionitis is infection of the amniotic fluid, membranes, placenta, and/or decidua. Diagnosis of clinical chorioamnionitis usually involves maternal fever in association with 2 of the following criteria: maternal tachycardia, fetal tachycardia, uterine tenderness, and foul odor of the amniotic fluid.[20] Other infectious causes of maternal fever to consider include urinary tract infection and respiratory infection.

The association of maternal fever and epidural analgesia has raised concerns about the increased risk of maternal infection with epidural catheter placement. Dashe and colleagues[15] studied the relationship between placental inflammation and maternal fever. They prospectively studied placentas of 149 patients, 54% of whom received epidural analgesia. Placental inflammation was greater in the epidural group (61% vs 36%). Maternal fever and placental inflammation also was significantly more common in the epidural analgesia group (35% vs 17%), although maternal fever was not increased in patients with epidural analgesia who did not have placental inflammation (11% vs 9%). Women with epidural analgesia had a longer duration of ruptured membranes as well as duration of labor, both of which are known risk factors for intrauterine infection. They concluded that epidural analgesia is associated with maternal fever only in the presence of histologic chorioamnionitis, thus the fever is a result of the infection and not the epidural analgesia.

Vallejo and colleagues[21] also studied the association between epidural analgesia and chorioamnionitis. They retrospectively compared 3 groups: (1) parturients with clinical chorioamnionitis and no epidural analgesia, (2) parturients with chorioamnionitis who had epidural analgesia, and (3) parturients who had epidural analgesia and no evidence of infection. Clinical diagnosis of chorioamnionitis was confirmed by histologic examination. Incidence of fever in patients with chorioamnionitis and no epidural analgesia (group 1) was 100%. Patients with epidural analgesia and chorioamnionitis (group 2) also had a fever 100% of the time. Patients with epidural analgesia and no evidence of chorioamnionitis (group 3) had an incidence of only 1%. These results confirmed the results of Dashe and colleagues[15] and confirmed that epidural analgesia was not associated with fever in the absence of chorioamnionitis.

Altered Thermoregulation

Another possible mechanism for maternal temperature increase during labor is altered thermoregulation. Heat balance is determined by metabolic heat production and cutaneous heat loss. Normal metabolic activities of the body, including labor, result in heat production. The hypothalamus then triggers processes such as vasodilation, sweating, and hyperventilation to promote heat loss.

In general, epidural analgesia initially causes a decrease in core temperatures primarily by redistribution of body heat from the core to the periphery and then a net heat loss to the environment.[13] This effect is then balanced by epidural analgesia decreasing the thermoregulatory threshold for shivering by blocking cold afferent thermal inputs from the anesthetized portion of the body, and shivering increases heat production. In addition, the sympathectomy from epidural analgesia inhibits sweating. Because sweating decreases core temperatures by increasing evaporative loss, epidural analgesia may increase core temperature.[22]

Labor is a known metabolic state that has been associated with a temporary increase in intrauterine temperatures, in part because of increased oxygen consumption with uterine and skeletal muscle contraction. Nulliparous patients have a greater increase in temperature than multiparous patients.[23] The increased intrauterine temperatures combined with the inability to dissipate heat through sweating may account for the associated temperature increase.

In addition, patients who do not receive analgesia during labor tend to hyperventilate and have increased sweating and heat loss resulting in lower core body temperatures.[24] By providing effective analgesia, the degree of hyperventilation and heat loss decreases with a potential for increased core temperatures.[11]

Fusi and colleagues[6] and Yancey and colleagues[10] both showed a temperature increase in parturients after epidural placement but did not find any evidence of infection in either the parturients or neonates. They both suggest that, because infectious causes are unlikely, temperature increases may be attributed to altered mechanisms of heat dissipation.

De Orange and colleagues[16] noted a significant increase in median maternal temperature as early as 1 hour after CSE, which disappeared after 6 hours of labor, in contrast with the nonpharmacologic group. Despite the increased incidence of fever, no cases of maternal infection were found. The investigators concluded that, with CSE, the increase in fever was not caused by infection but possibly by an alteration in maternal thermoregulation.

Mantha and colleagues[18] found that intermittent epidural injections seem to protect against intrapartum fever in the first 4 hours of labor analgesia as compared to continuous infusion. Because no differences were seen in neonatal sepsis evaluation, they thought that infection was an unlikely cause. Intermittent partial recovery of heat loss mechanisms between injections may be an explanation.

The effects of shivering after epidural placement on heat production and possible maternal fevers have also been considered. Camann and colleagues[14] found no evidence of infection despite an increase in maternal temperature in patients receiving epidural analgesia. Shivering occurred rarely in their study.

Gleeson and colleagues[25] found that clinical fever occurred 3 times more often in women who shivered compared with those who did not after epidural placement. Laboring patients who shivered after epidural administration also developed fever as early as 1 hour after placement as opposed to greater than 4 hours for those who did not shiver.

Inflammation

The theory of noninfectious inflammation with epidural analgesia as an explanation for maternal temperature increases has also been proposed.

Negishi and colleagues[26] determined that opioids inhibit an increase in temperature when given intravenously. Fever was induced in 8 volunteers by giving them intravenous interleukin (IL) - 2 on 4 different study days. Each volunteer was randomly assigned on each study day to either a control, when no opioid or epidural analgesia was given, epidural analgesia with ropivacaine and fentanyl, epidural analgesia with ropivacaine alone, or intravenous fentanyl. Fentanyl caused a decrease in core temperature on the control day and on the intravenous fentanyl day, whereas epidural analgesia did not inhibit a febrile response. These results support the conclusion that epidural analgesia is associated with inflammation and not necessarily infection.

Goetzl and colleagues[27] performed a secondary analysis of a study that prospectively randomized nulliparous women with epidural analgesia to either acetaminophen or placebo. Maternal serum and cord blood samples were obtained. Maternal IL-6 was higher in patients who were febrile. In addition, neonates born to febrile mothers had a higher level of IL-6. The increased levels of inflammatory cytokines suggest an inflammatory mechanism for the fever.

Because fever may be associated with negative consequences, prophylactic treatment of fever may reduce the negative impact of maternal fever. Goetzl and colleagues[28] prospectively randomized 42 nulliparous patients receiving epidural analgesia to acetaminophen or placebo. Treatment with acetaminophen had no effect on maternal temperature over time. The overall incidence of fever (23.8%) was the same in both groups. As part of the study protocol, all neonates had a blood culture done, all of which were negative. No difference was found between placental inflammation or funisitis in either group.

Because acetaminophen, which acts at the hypothalamic thermoregulatory set point, had no effect on temperature, it seems that maternal fever may not be a result of thermoregulatory changes but rather an inflammatory response.

Riley and colleagues[29] performed an observational analysis of placental cultures and serum cytokine levels in 200 parturients. Women self-selected the type of analgesia. Women with epidural analgesia were more likely to be febrile but not more likely to have a placental infection. Rate of infection was similar regardless of maternal fever. Admission IL-6 levels greater than 11 pg/mL were associated with increased incidence of fevers in the epidural group. At delivery, women who had epidural analgesia, regardless of fever, had higher IL-6 levels than those who did not. This study supports the theory that fever is associated with an inflammatory mechanism.

RISK FACTORS

Risk factors for developing fever include nulliparity, long duration of labor, prolonged rupture of membranes, induction of labor, and dysfunctional labor. Many of theses risk factors are the same for intrapartum infection, including nulliparity, induction of labor, internal monitoring, more vaginal examinations, longer labor, and longer duration of ruptured membranes. These factors also often result in a request for epidural analgesia. As a result, it is difficult to separate an increase in maternal temperature caused by epidural analgesia from increased maternal temperatures caused by risk factors that predispose patients to desire epidural analgesia.

Herbst and colleagues[7] retrospectively found that nulliparity, duration of labor, and epidural analgesia were independent risk factors for fever. Other significant factors included rupture of membranes for longer than 24 hours, a temperature at the upper range of normal on arrival, and a long interval from arrival to established labor.

Froelich and colleagues[4] prospectively studied the time course of maternal temperature and other factors that are associated with an increase in maternal temperature in women undergoing induction of labor. In the 81 women enrolled, they found a significant linear trend in temperature of 0.017°C/h. Higher temperature increases were associated with higher body mass index and longer duration of ruptured membranes to delivery. Temperature slopes before and after initiation of epidural analgesia were determined and then tested to establish whether the slope of the temperature changes was different from zero. The 95% confidence interval was −0.0068 - 0.00338, which indicated that epidural analgesia did not affect maternal temperature. Lieberman and colleague[8] found that the incidence of fever increased with longer labors from 7% with labors of less than 6 hours to 36% for those greater than 18 hours. In the study by Philip and colleagues,[12] labor was significantly longer in women who were febrile regardless of parity or type of analgesia. Nulliparity and prolonged labor were independent risk factors for development of fever. Gonen and colleagues[9] determined that epidural analgesia duration correlated with maternal fever, which was independent of labor duration. The rate of fever increased with the duration of epidural analgesia.

CONSEQUENCES

Maternal fever has significant consequences for both the mother and fetus. Maternal effects of increased temperature include tachycardia, increased cardiac output, oxygen consumption, and catecholamine production.[30] Most laboring women are otherwise healthy and tolerate these changes well. Maternal temperature increase has also been shown to affect delivery plans.

Lieberman and colleagues[31] studied the effects of maternal temperature increase on rates of cesarean and assisted vaginal delivery. More than 1200 low-risk term nulliparous women who were afebrile on admission were analyzed. Even after controlling for birth weight, length of labor, and use of epidural analgesia, women with temperatures greater than 37.5°C had a 2-fold higher risk of both cesarean and assisted vaginal delivery. In addition, febrile women were more likely to have antibiotic exposure, usually to treat presumed chorioamnionitis or for surgical prophylaxis.[32]

There is always concern that, in addition to maternal effects, intrapartum fever will cause adverse outcomes in the neonate. Maternal infection in particular is of great concern because sepsis in the newborn may result. Even when the cause is noninfectious, there are concerns that increased maternal temperatures can have adverse fetal and neonatal outcomes. Fetal effects of maternal fever are thought to be caused by transfer of heat to the fetus, causing hyperthermia.

In the 1970s, Morishima and colleagues[33] studied the consequences of maternal hyperthermia in 23 pregnant baboons. Maternal temperatures were artificially increased by radiant warming up to 41 to 42°C to determine fetal outcomes in the absence of infection. These extreme temperatures were associated with increased uterine activity, acidosis, and hemodynamic instability in both mother and fetus. In addition, late decelerations were more common than during normal temperature conditions. Although both mothers and fetuses had adverse outcomes, these extreme temperatures are rarely encountered in clinical practice.

Harris and colleagues[34] also conducted an animal study in the 1970s with pregnant ewes that developed fevers after injection of a bacterial pyrogen. Maternal and fetal temperatures increased in parallel and outcomes were measured as temperatures increased. During the fever, fetal heart rate variability was seen but changes in oxygenation or acid/base status were not observed.

Lieberman and colleagues[31] performed several studies investigating neonatal outcomes after maternal fever. One such study showed that intrapartum fever was associated with greater neonatal sepsis evaluations as well as neonatal antibiotic administration.[31] Thirty-four percent of the sepsis work-ups were in patients who had received epidural analgesia during labor versus 10% who did not get an epidural catheter. Infants whose mothers had epidural analgesia were 4 times more likely to receive antibiotics. These infants were also 3 times more likely to receive antibiotics for greater than 3 days (odds ratio = 3.3). These results generated concern in the medical community and the media because of the conclusion that epidural analgesia increased the risk of neonatal sepsis evaluations. Goetzl and colleagues[35] studied more than 1100 women who were afebrile (temperature <38.0°C) throughout labor and noted an increase in neonatal sepsis work-up in women with epidural analgesia but no increase in the incidence of neonatal sepsis.

Greenwell and colleagues[36] retrospectively studied neonatal outcomes in infants born to low-risk parturients who either had epidural analgesia or not. Maternal temperature greater than 38.0°C was more prevalent in the epidural analgesia group. There was no difference in outcome in the absence of increased maternal temperature. A significant linear trend was noted between maximum maternal temperature and adverse neonatal outcomes. Infants born to mothers with fever greater than 38.0°C had a 2-fold to 6-fold increased risk for adverse outcomes.

Another study by Lieberman and colleagues[37] involved 1218 women and compared neonatal outcomes in febrile versus nonfebrile mothers. The neonatal outcomes included Apgar scores, resuscitation, hypotonia, seizures, and the need for oxygen therapy in the nursery. Compared with the afebrile group, the 10% of women with temperatures greater than 38.0°C were more likely to have neonates with low 1-minute Apgar scores (<7), with hypotonia requiring bag mask resuscitation, and with oxygen therapy in the nursery. There also was a slightly higher rate of seizures in the febrile group. By 5 minutes, less than 1% of neonates had Apgars less than 7.

In the previous study, the number of neonatal seizures was small, so Lieberman and colleagues[38] conducted a case-control study from a neonatal database to further investigate the association of maternal fever in labor with unexplained neonatal seizures among term infants. Thirty-eight term infants with unexplained seizures were compared with 152 controls. The infants with seizures were more than 3 times more likely to be born to mothers who were febrile during labor. None of the infants with seizure had documentation of neonatal infection.

The association of adverse neurologic outcomes and maternal fever has garnered much attention over the years. Neonates born to mothers with chorioamnionitis are thought to be at highest risk. However, even isolated fever without chorioamnionitis seems to have an increased risk. Blume and colleagues[39] performed a case-control study of 1060 term newborns with diagnosis of encephalopathy and compared them with 5330 unaffected controls. Isolated intrapartum fever was associated with 3.1-fold increased risk and chorioamnionitis was associated with a 5.4-fold increased risk of encephalopathy.

Impey and colleagues[40] performed a prospective cohort study of nearly 5000 low-risk women, looking for differences in neonatal outcome between women who developed a temperature greater than 37.5°C during labor and those who did not. All women were afebrile at the diagnosis of labor. The maternal fever group had a statistically significant higher rate of neonatal encephalopathy, with an odds ratio of 4.72. They also noted a higher base deficit and increased neonatal unit admissions. Several other studies also noted an association between maternal chorioamnionitis and cerebral palsy.[41]

In addition to immediate neonatal consequences, several long-term outcomes have been associated with maternal fever. Dammann and colleagues[42] showed a statistically significant association between lower nonverbal intelligence scores and maternal fever. Of the 294 cases analyzed, there was nearly a 4-fold increase in low nonverbal intelligence scores at age 9 years when maternal temperature was greater than 38.5°C at birth. Low scores were considered to be greater than 2 standard deviations less than the mean. Maternal fever may also have some link to schizophrenia, autism, and Parkinson disease.[30]

SUMMARY

Epidural analgesia has been associated with increased maternal temperatures and fevers in laboring women compared with those who use other forms of analgesia. The mechanism for this fever is unlikely to be of infectious origin. The underlying cause is unclear, although it seems to be a combination of altered thermoregulation and inflammation after epidural analgesia. Other risk factors for maternal fever, including nulliparity, prolonged or dysfunctional labor, and prolonged rupture of membranes, increase the need for epidural analgesia. These risk factors also may explain the strong association between maternal fever and epidural analgesia. The consequences of epidural-associated maternal fever on neonatal outcomes require further investigation. There may be an increase in sepsis work-ups in light of the fever, but it is unclear whether there is any associated neonatal brain injury. Further research is needed to investigate the causes and consequences of fever accompanying epidural analgesia during labor.

REFERENCES

1. Acker DB, Schulman EB, Ransil BJ, et al. The normal parturient's admission temperature. Am J Obstet Gynecol 1987;157:308–11.
2. Bartholomew ML, Ashkin E, Schiffman A, et al. Maternal temperature variation during parturition. Obstet Gynecol 2002;100:642–7.
3. Schouten FD, Wolf H, Smith BJ, et al. Maternal temperature during labour. BJOG 2008;115:1131–7.
4. Froelich MA, Esame A, Zhang K, et al. What factors affect intrapartum maternal temperature? A prospective cohort study: maternal intrapartum temperature. Anesthesiology 2012;117:302–8.
5. Banerjee S, Cashman P, Yentis SM, et al. Maternal temperature monitoring during labor: concordance and variability among monitoring sites. Obstet Gynecol 2004; 103:287–93.
6. Fusi L, Steer PJ, Maresh MJ, et al. Maternal pyrexia associated with the use of epidural analgesia in labour. Lancet 1989;1:1250–2.
7. Herbst A, Wolner-Hanssen P, Ingemarsson I. Risk factors for fever in labor. Obstet Gynecol 1995;86:790–4.
8. Lieberman E, Lang JM, Frigoletto F Jr, et al. Epidural analgesia, intrapartum fever, and neonatal sepsis evaluation. Pediatrics 1997;99:415–9.
9. Gonen R, Korobochka R, Degani S, et al. Association between epidural analgesia and intrapartum fever. Am J Perinatol 2000;17(3):127–30.
10. Yancey MK, Zhang J, Schwarz J, et al. Labor epidural analgesia and intrapartum maternal hyperthermia. Obstet Gynecol 2001;98:763–70.
11. Macaulay JH, Bond K, Steer PJ. Epidural analgesia in labor and fetal hyperthermia. Obstet Gynecol 1992;80:665–9.
12. Philip J, Alexander JM, Sharma SK, et al. Epidural analgesia during labor and maternal fever. Anesthesiology 1999;90:1271–5.
13. Matsukawa T, Sessler DI, Christenson R, et al. Heat flow and distribution during epidural anesthesia. Anesthesiology 1995;83:961–7.
14. Camann WR, Horveth LA, Hughes N, et al. Maternal temperature regulation during extradural analgesia for labour. Br J Anaesth 1991;67:565–8.
15. Dashe JS, Rogers BB, McIntire DD, et al. Epidural analgesia and intrapartum fever: placental findings. Obstet Gynecol 1999;93:341–4.
16. De Orange FA, Passini R, Amorim M, et al. Combined spinal and epidural anaesthesia and maternal intrapartum temperature during vaginal delivery: a randomized clinical trial. Br J Anaesth 2011;107:762–8.
17. Sharma SK, Alexander JM, Messick G, et al. Cesarean delivery: a randomized trial of epidural analgesia versus intravenous meperidine analgesia during labor in nulliparous women. Anesthesiology 2002;96:546–51.

18. Mantha VR, Vallejo MC, Ramesh V, et al. The incidence of maternal fever during labor is less with intermittent than with continuous epidural analgesia: a randomized controlled trial. Int J Obstet Anesth 2008;17:123–9.
19. Vinson DC, Thomas R, Kiser T. Association between epidural analgesia during labor and fever. J Fam Pract 1993;36:617–22.
20. Tita AT, Andrews WW. Diagnosis and management of clinical chorioamnionitis. Clin Perinatol 2010;37:339–54.
21. Vallejo MC, Kaul B, Adler LJ, et al. Chorioamnionitis, not epidural analgesia, is associated with maternal fever during labour. Can J Anaesth 2001;48:1122–6.
22. Glosten B, Savage M, Rooke GA, et al. Epidural anesthesia and the thermoregulatory response to hyperthermia – preliminary observations in volunteer subjects. Acta Anaesthesiol Scand 1998;42:442–6.
23. Marx GF, Loew DA. Tympanic temperature during labour and parturition. Br J Anaesth 1975;47:600–2.
24. Goodlin RC, Chapin JW. Determinants of maternal temperature during labor. Am J Obstet Gynecol 1982;143:97–103.
25. Gleeson NC, Nolan KM, Ford MR. Temperature, labour, and epidural analgesia. Lancet 1989;2:861–2.
26. Negishi C, Lenhardt R, Ozaki M, et al. Opioids inhibit febrile responses in humans, whereas epidural analgesia does not: an explanation for hyperthermia during epidural analgesia. Anesthesiology 2001;94:218–22.
27. Goetzl L, Evans T, Rivers J, et al. Elevated maternal and fetal serum interleukin-6 levels are associated with epidural fever. Am J Obstet Gynecol 2002;187:834–8.
28. Goetzl L, Rivers J, Evans T, et al. Prophylactic acetaminophen does not prevent epidural fever in nulliparous women: a double-blind placebo-controlled trial. J Perinatol 2004;24:471–5.
29. Riley LE, Celi AC, Onderdonk AB, et al. Association of epidural-related fever and noninfectious inflammation in term labor. Obstet Gynecol 2011;117:588–95.
30. Segal S. Labor epidural analgesia and maternal fever. Anesth Analg 2010;111:1467–75.
31. Lieberman E, Cohen A, Lang J, et al. Maternal intrapartum temperature elevation as a risk factor for cesarean delivery and assisted vaginal delivery. Am J Public Health 1999;89:506–10.
32. Goetzl L, Cohen A, Frigoletto F Jr, et al. Maternal epidural analgesia and rates of maternal antibiotic treatment in a low-risk nulliparous population. J Perinatol 2003;23:457–61.
33. Morishima HO, Glaser B, Niemann WH, et al. Increased uterine activity and fetal deterioration during maternal hyperthermia. Am J Obstet Gynecol 1975;121:531–8.
34. Harris WH, Pittman QJ, Veale WL, et al. Cardiovascular effects of fever in the ewe and fetal lamb. Am J Obstet Gynecol 1977;128:262–5.
35. Goetzl L, Cohen A, Frigoletto F Jr, et al. Maternal epidural use and neonatal sepsis evaluation in afebrile mothers. Pediatrics 2001;108:1099–102.
36. Greenwell EA, Wyshak G, Ringer SA, et al. Intrapartum temperature elevation, epidural use, and adverse outcome in term infants. Pediatrics 2012;129:e447–54.
37. Lieberman E, Lang L, Richardson DK, et al. Intrapartum maternal fever and neonatal outcome. Pediatrics 2000;105:8–13.
38. Lieberman E, Eichenwald E, Mathur G, et al. Intrapartum fever and unexplained seizures in term infants. Pediatrics 2000;106:983–8.

39. Blume HK, Li CI, Loch CM, et al. Intrapartum fever and chorioamnionitis as risks for encephalopathy in term newborns: a case-control study. Dev Med Child Neurol 2008;50:19–24.
40. Impey L, Greenwood C, MacQuillan K, et al. Fever in labour and neonatal encephalopathy: a prospective cohort study. BJOG 2001;108:594–7.
41. Grether JK, Nelson KB. Maternal infection and cerebral palsy in infants of normal birth weight. JAMA 1997;278:207–11.
42. Dammann O, Drescher J, Veelken N. Maternal fever at birth and non-verbal intelligence at age 9 years in preterm infants. Dev Med Child Neurol 2003;45:148–51.

Neurologic Complications of Neuraxial Anesthesia

Elaine Pages-Arroyo, MD[a],*, May C.M. Pian-Smith, MD, MS[b]

KEYWORDS

- Spinal • Epidural • Headache • Neuraxial anesthesia complications • Neurology
- Obstetrics • Peripheral neuropathy • Regional anesthesia

KEY POINTS

- Proper technique with neuraxial procedures minimizes the risk of complications such as dural puncture, pneumocephalus, meningitis, direct spinal cord injury, and arachnoiditis.
- Serious complications are truly rare, but need to be diagnosed and managed in a timely manner.
- If postdural puncture headache is suspected, immediate conservative treatment should be initiated and invasive treatment considered if headache persists; further neurologic evaluation should be pursued for refractory cases.
- 20% Intralipid emulsion should be available for the treatment of local anesthetic toxicity syndrome in any location where epidural anesthesia is performed.
- Patients with bleeding/coagulation concerns are at highest risk of developing an epidural hematoma.
- Cord ischemia, epidural abscess, and arachnoiditis are rare but potentially catastrophic complications of neuraxial procedures; neurosurgery consultation should be made immediately.
- Nonspecific back pain may develop in 44% of the pregnant population, regardless of the use of neuraxial analgesia/anesthesia.
- Peripheral nerve injuries are common complications of childbirth trauma that are frequently and erroneously attributed to the use of neuraxial techniques.

NEUROLOGIC COMPLICATIONS RELATED TO THE BRAIN
Postdural Puncture Headache

Etiology and symptoms
A postdural puncture headache (PDPH) may occur after a spinal anesthetic or after inadvertent dural puncture during epidural catheter placement. Incidence of inadvertent dural puncture during epidural catheter placement is approximately 1%, and is associated with an 80%[1] (range 45%–80%)[2] risk of PDPH. After a spinal neuraxial

[a] Department of Anesthesia, Brigham and Women's Hospital, 75 Francis Street, Boston, MA 02115, USA; [b] Department of Anesthesia, Critical Care and Pain Medicine, Massachusetts General Hospital, 55 Fruit Street, Boston, MA 02114-2696, USA
* Corresponding author.
E-mail address: emarie27@gmail.com

Anesthesiology Clin 31 (2013) 571–594
http://dx.doi.org/10.1016/j.anclin.2013.05.001
1932-2275/13/$ – see front matter Published by Elsevier Inc.

anesthesiology.theclinics.com

Box 1
International Headache Society definition of postdural puncture headache

Onset within 5 days after dural puncture

Worsening within 15 minutes after sitting or standing

Improves within 15 minutes after lying down

With at least 1 of the following:

- Neck stiffness

- Tinnitus

- Hypacusia

- Photophobia

- Nausea

In 95% of cases, headache resolves spontaneously within 1 week or within 48 hours after effective treatment of spinal fluid leak, usually with an epidural blood patch

Data from International Headache Society. The international classification of headache disorders. 2nd edition. Oxford (UK): Blackwell Publishing; 2004.

Box 2
Symptomatology associated with postdural puncture headache

Frontal or occipital location of headache

Neck stiffness (43%)[1]

Worsening symptoms when sitting up or standing versus when supine

Ocular (13%) and auditory (12%) symptoms[1]

Box 3
Differential diagnosis of persistent postpartum headache

Nonspecific headache

Postdural puncture headache

Preeclampsia/hypertension

Migraines

Sinusitis

Pneumocephalus

Intracranial bleed

- Subdural

- Subarachnoid

- Intracerebral

Meningitis

Cerebral vein thrombosis

Cerebral infarction/ischemia

Pseudotumor cerebri

Intracranial tumor

Table 1
Treatment of postdural puncture headache

Conservative: Initial Therapy	Invasive: Epidural Blood Patch; After Failed Conservative Therapy

Psychological support
  Expressing empathy for patient
  Renewing commitment to ongoing care
Horizontal position
  Alleviates symptoms in the short term
  Decreases ongoing CSF leak more long
  term
	Prophylactic blood patch (before onset of
	  headache): high failure risk[2,4]
	Preferably performed after 24 h for more
	  effective results[5]

Hydration[6]
  Supports choroid plexus production of CSF
  Enhances intravascular volume
  Caffeinated beverages[6] (used for many
  years despite clear evidence of its
  efficacy[1])
	Usual technique as when placing an epidural
	  needle; some practitioners use a loss of
	  resistance to saline technique to minimize
	  the risk of pneumocephalus
	An average of 20 mL of the patient's blood,
	  collected with sterile technique, is
	  injected[7]

Pharmacologic treatment
  Analgesics: acetaminophen, NSAIDs,
  Fioricet
  Sumatriptan: of controversial value
  according to studies[1]
  Adrenocorticotropic hormone[4]: not
  recommended as first-line therapy but
  may be considered for persistent cases
  not amenable to epidural blood patch[2]
  Gabapentin, methylergonovine, and
  hydrocortisone: reports of use but need
  further study related to efficacy and
  safety for the treatment of PDPH[2]
	Injection is stopped if the patient complains
	  of back pain or neurologic symptoms of
	  the lower extremities
	Advisable to go one level lower than initial
	  neuraxial block because 70% of the
	  injected blood will spread cephalad[2]
	When performed later than 24 h after wet
	  tap has success rate of 70%–97%.[2]
	Obstetric studies showed that
	  approximately 30% of patients would
	  present with recurrence of headache
	  necessitating a second blood patch.[8] Usual
	  practice is to allow for an interval of 24 h
	  between repeat blood patches
	There are few cases whereby a third EBP has
	  been performed for a selected group of
	  patients with recurrent PDPH using CT
	  guidance.[9] However, complications such as
	  permanent paralysis and cauda equina
	  syndrome, pneumocephalus, back pain,
	  radicular pain, epidural abscess, and facial
	  nerve paralysis have been reported.
	  Repeated injections of blood into the
	  epidural space may potentially lead to
	  fibrosis and obliteration of the epidural
	  space.[10,11] Mass effect as a result of blood
	  may also cause spinal cord and nerve root
	  compression
	Patient and caretakers should be advised to
	  seek attention for worsening headache or
	  signs and symptoms of epidural hematoma
	  or abscess

Abbreviations: CSF, cerebrospinal fluid; CT, computed tomography; EBP, epidural blood patch; NSAIDs, nonsteroidal anti-inflammatory drugs; PDPH, postdural puncture headache.

technique the rate of PDPH is reportedly 1.5% to 11.2%, depending on the needle size and type[2] and patient characteristics. Short-beveled Quinke needles cause PDPH more commonly than small-gauge pencil-point needles, and patients younger than 45 years and pregnant women are at higher risk of PDPH.[2] PDPH is caused by leakage of cerebrospinal fluid (CSF) through the dural hole, leading to relative intracranial hypotension and traction of the meninges and meningeal vessels (**Boxes 1** and **2**).

Occasionally, PDPH may persist for months, with a blood patch (at least at 12 months) being successful.[3] If headache persists despite therapy, other causes should be investigated (**Box 3**).

Diagnostic tests

The diagnosis of PDPH is primarily based on clinical presentation and is strengthened by a history or suspicion of dural puncture. Twenty-six percent of accidental dural punctures are unrecognized at the time of the procedure and first present as PDPH in the early puerperium.[3] The diagnosis is further supported by provocative testing, such as worsening of symptoms when the patient is deliberately moved from supine to upright positions.

Treatment

Early treatment is indicated to avoid immobility and depression of the patient and minimize interference with maternal newborn bonding. Early and effective treatment also minimizes the risk of rare but potential complications such as hearing loss, subdural hematoma, or dural sinus thrombosis (**Table 1**).

Subdural Hematomas

Etiology and symptoms

Intracranial subdural hematoma is a rare complication of neuraxial anesthetics in pregnant patients, and its incidence is unknown.[12] A recent review of the literature reports 25 cases of subdural hematoma after spinal anesthesia, and 21 cases after accidental dural puncture with an epidural needle.[13] The bleeding results from CSF leaks and decreased intracranial pressure (ICP). CSF leakage is further accentuated by maternal Valsalva during labor and delivery.[12] Initially decreased ICP causes traction on the bridging veins, which may bleed, causing intracranial hemorrhage. Subsequently, signs of increased ICP may manifest after there is significant bleeding (**Box 4**).

Diagnostic tests

Delayed diagnosis is a challenge with subdural hematomas in patients with PDPH.[13] The physician should have a high index of suspicion when there is a change in headache characteristics from postural to nonpostural or, when a PDPH persists despite more than 1 blood patch. The diagnosis is made by computed tomography (CT) or

---

Box 4
Signs of increased intracranial pressure

- Nonpostural headache
- Convulsions
- Hemiplegia
- Disorientation
- Somnolence
- Vomiting

magnetic resonance imaging (MRI). A CT scan is usually the first modality to be used because it easily detects acute hemorrhages and is more readily available than an MRI. On CT imaging, an acute subdural bleed will appear as a crescent-shaped collection with increased attenuation. The hemorrhage will become isoattenuated with CSF as the lesion becomes more chronic in nature. The bleeding may be accompanied by radiologic findings of intracranial hypotension such as pachymeningeal enhancement, sagging of the brain, and low-lying cerebellar tonsils.[14] On the other hand, MRI is more specific and sensitive, and identifies small hemorrhages (also identified as crescent-shaped collections) that can be missed otherwise. The detection rate for subdural hemorrhage is more than 95% on the T2-weighted modality, which enhances tissue differentiation.[15–17]

Treatment

Management is conservative or surgical, depending on the size of the bleed. Small bleeds that resolve may be followed up with regular management. An early epidural blood patch may prevent formation of a subdural hematoma by stopping ongoing leakage of CSF and significant intracranial hypotension.[13]

Pneumocephalus

Etiology and symptoms

The entry of air into the intracranial cavity is a rare complication of neuraxial techniques.[18] When performing placement of an epidural catheter with the loss of resistance to air, air may enter the intraparenchymal, subarachnoid, intraventricular, subdural, or epidural spaces. Like a space-occupying lesion, it can be associated with neurologic symptoms.[2] Pneumocephalus can also occur during subarachnoid injections (**Table 2**).

Table 2	
Symptoms associated with pneumocephalus	
More common	Headache (usually abrupt onset immediately after neuraxial technique[19])
Less common	Nausea and vomiting
	Tinnitus
	Blurry vision
	Seizures
	Dizziness
	Depressed level of consciousness

Diagnostic tests

Diagnosis can be made by plain radiographs or CT scan.[2] Most commonly a CT scan is performed, demonstrating air-filled cavities in the subarachnoid space in different areas of the brain such as in the suprasellar area, optic chiasm, and frontal, temporal, and parietal lobes. As with the diagnosis of pneumothorax, significant quantities of air over the frontal convexities produce the "Mount Fuji" sign, and multiple scattered air bubbles throughout the cisterns are known as the air-bubble sign.[20]

Differential diagnosis

The headache caused by pneumocephalus mimics a PDPH headache[2] in that it can get worse while the patient is sitting up or standing. The differential should include PDPH, meningitis, and chemical arachnoiditis.[2] Intracranial hemorrhage is also on the differential of new-onset headache after a neuraxial technique, and can be differentiated by CT.

Treatment

Standard management is conservative with reassurance, bed rest, and analgesics (opioids, nonsteroidal anti-inflammatory drugs [NSAIDs]). Ventilatory support may be necessary in severe cases. The literature reports spontaneous reabsorption rates from 24 hours to 1 week, with most patients recovering without any neurologic sequelae. Presence of persistent lethargy, confusion, headache, slow arousal, hemiparesis, or hemiplegia is concerning, and may necessitate emergency surgical treatment.

As an adjuvant to standard conservative treatment, high-concentration inspired oxygen has been reported to accelerate the reabsorption of intracranial air. In 1996 Dexter and Reasoner published evidence that, based on mathematical model predictions, a fraction of inspired oxygen (Fio_2) of 0.4 to 1.0 for 1 to 2 weeks would decrease the time needed for a pneumocephalus to be reabsorbed.[21] A recent prospective study of postcraniotomy patients demonstrated statistically significant differences in rates of pneumocephalus absorption between a control group receiving room air and a group receiving supplemental oxygen through a non-rebreather mask.[22] Such therapy needs to be given with appropriate caution: air in the brain cavity may be increased and may even result in a tension pneumocephalus when hyperbaric oxygen therapy is used.[23–25]

Meningitis

Etiology and symptoms

Although it is an infrequent complication of neuraxial anesthesia techniques,[13] meningitis with viral, bacterial, and fungal causes has been reported.[26] The most common causative organisms come from the oral and nasal passages of health care providers.[13,26,27] Species of the *Streptococcus* and *Pseudomonas* have been identified in CSF cultures.[26] Infectious organisms also originate from contaminated equipment and patients' skin and blood.[27] Additional risk factors include vaginal infections, bacteremia, poor aseptic techniques, and immune system compromise. Incidence has been reported to be approximately 1 in 39,000 neuraxial blocks.[13]

Symptoms are frequently confused with manifestations of PDPH.[1] Signs and symptoms can manifest hours or a few days after the anesthetic (**Box 5**).[26]

Diagnostic tests

A comprehensive evaluation when meningitis is suspected includes a medical history, physical examination, and laboratory workup such as complete blood count, CSF analysis, and blood cultures. Examination of the CSF is the basis for the diagnosis of central nervous system infections. The classic CSF findings will vary according to the origin of the infection (**Table 3**).

Box 5
Typical symptomatology of Meningitis

- Headache
- Fever
- Nausea and vomiting
- Malaise
- Altered mental status
- Irritability
- Neck stiffness
- Back pain

Table 3
Characteristic findings of CSF analysis for meningitis

Etiology	Cells/mL	% PMN	Glucose	Protein (mg/dL)
Bacterial	500–10,000	>90	<40 mg/dL	<150
Aseptic	10–500	<50	Normal	<100
Viral	0–1000	<50	Normal	<100

Abbreviation: PMN, polymorphonuclear cells.

Treatment

The mainstay of treatment is antibiotic therapy, which should not be delayed for definitive diagnosis.[13,26] Broad-spectrum antibiotics are initiated while the causative organism is identified or its sensitivities are established.

Local Anesthetic Toxicity

Symptoms

Local anesthetic toxicity syndrome (LATS) has been reported in the obstetric population after accidental intravascular injection.[28–30] The onset and spectrum of toxicity vary depending on several factors: type of local anesthetic used, speed of injection, and type of regional block being performed. Because it is dose dependent, it is rare with spinal[13] neuraxial techniques, but can occur with large volumes of anesthetics with intended epidural blocks. Incidence is approximately 1 in every 10,000 epidural blocks.[31] Of all local anesthetics, bupivacaine is associated with the highest toxicity, owing to its prolonged and high affinity for sodium channels in neurons and cardiac cells (**Table 4**).

Diagnosis

LATS is diagnosed based on clinical history and symptoms. Serum levels of local anesthetic can be assayed, but supportive and definitive treatment should not be delayed (**Tables 5 and 6**).

Management

Prevention of LATS is facilitated by aspirating the epidural catheter for the presence of blood, and administering the local anesthetic in incremental doses instead of a single large dose. Careful observation of the patient after bolusing the catheter is prudent. Early recognition and early treatment are essential for patient survival. Administration of lipid emulsion has become the gold standard of therapy, although an animal study suggests that coadministration of high-dose epinephrine during resuscitations may interfere with the efficacy of lipid rescue.[33,34] It has been suggested that in humans,

Table 4
Signs and symptoms of local anesthetic toxicity

Early	Late
Tinnitus	Seizures
Metallic taste	Loss of consciousness
Diplopia	Further neurologic deterioration and cardiac toxicity leading to:
Circumoral paresthesia	Respiratory arrest
Agitation	Cardiovascular collapse
Confusion	Hypotension
	Arrhythmias
	Cardiac arrest

Data from Di Gregorio G, Neal JM, Rosenquist RW, et al. Clinical presentation of local anesthetic systemic toxicity: a review of published cases, 1979 to 2009. Reg Anesth Pain Med 2010;35(2):181–7.

Table 5
Differential diagnosis of local anesthetic toxicity syndrome

Obstetric Complications	Anesthetic Complications	Others
Eclampsia Amniotic fluid embolism	Total spinal anaphylaxis Local anesthetic vascular injection Overdose of local anesthetic Reaction to vasoconstrictors	Vasovagal reaction Other causes of cardiac compromise: myocardial infarction, pulmonary embolus, cardiomyopathy Other causes of seizure disorder: hypoglycemia, cerebrovascular accident Other causes of respiratory failure: magnesium toxicity

Table 6
Treatment of local anesthetic toxicity syndrome

General Considerations	Neurologic Manifestations	Cardiovascular Collapse	Lipid Emulsion Therapy[32]
Call for help Consider cardiopulmonary bypass	Control seizures: benzodiazepines preferred Protect the airway from aspiration Avoid hypoxia: ventilate patient with 100% Fio_2	Advanced cardiac life support	20% lipid emulsion: 20% soybean oil, 1.2% egg yolk phospholipids, 2.25% glycerin, water, and sodium hydroxide Bolus 1.5 mg/kg over 1 min Repeat bolus once or twice for persistent cardiovascular collapse Continuous intravenous infusion at 0.25 ml/kg/min Increase infusion to 0.5 ml/kg/min if hypotension is refractory Continue infusion for at least 10 min after obtaining circulatory stability

Data from Dillane D, Finucane BT. Local anesthetic systemic toxicity. Can J Anaesth 2010;57(4):36880.

the use of low-dose epinephrine (1–2.5 µg/kg) with the lipid emulsion may provide the most benefit.[28]

Changes in Mental Status Caused by High Intrathecal Block

Symptoms
A high or total intrathecal block most commonly presents when a large volume of local anesthetic is accidentally injected through a spinal catheter presumed to be in the epidural space, or when there is excessive cephalad spread of local anesthetics injected into the subarachnoid space. It also may occur when a spinal anesthetic is placed after an inadequate epidural block. Total intrathecal block occurs after anesthesia of the spinal cord, cervical spinal nerves, and brainstem.[13] The overall incidence of total spinal block is unknown,[13] although it contributed to 22 cases of obstetric cardiac arrest as reported by the 2007 Doctors Company review.[35] In 2009 the ASA Closed Claims report cited high spinals as the most concerning complication of neuraxial anesthesia in the United States: high spinals resulted in 15 lawsuits for maternal brain injury or death (**Box 6**).[36]

Box 6
Risk factors for a high or total subarachnoid block

- Obesity and pregnancy
  - Engorged epidural veins
  - Increased intra-abdominal pressure
  - Reduced size of subarachnoid space that favors cephalad spread of local anesthetics
- Fluid in epidural space from epidural infusion: further compresses the subarachnoid space
- Dose, volume, and baricity can affect spread

Table 7
Clinical manifestations of complete spinal block

Difficulty breathing and speaking	Pupillary dilation
Apnea	Loss of consciousness
Decreased oxygen saturation	Respiratory arrest
Nausea and vomiting	Hypotension
Anxiety/altered mental status	Bradycardia
Hand and arm dysesthesia or paralysis	Cardiovascular collapse/arrest
High sensory block	

Table 8
Differential diagnosis of complete spinal block

Respiratory depression	Pulmonary embolus
Hypotension	Amniotic fluid embolism
Drug overdose	Pulmonary edema
Anxiety, panic attack	Hypoglycemia
Seizures	Vascular injection of local anesthetics

Data from Chan SK, Karmakar MK, Chui PT. Local anesthesia outside the operating room. Hong Kong Med J 2002;8(2):106–13; and Lui KC, Chow YF. Safe use of local anaesthetics: prevention and management of systemic toxicity. Hong Kong Med J 2010;16(6):470–5.

Signs and symptoms usually manifest almost immediately after injection (**Tables 7 and 8**).

A high or total intrathecal block is a clinical diagnosis. The anesthesiologist must have a high index of suspicion and should initiate early supportive treatment. With early recognition and treatment, the onset of respiratory arrest and cardiovascular collapse may be avoided. The patient may be placed in the reverse Trendelenburg position to avoid further cephalad spread of hyperbaric anesthetic. Hypotension can be treated with fluid boluses as well as vasopressor medications. For bradycardia, atropine or epinephrine may be administered intravenously. Initiation of ventilatory support is vital, starting with supplemental oxygen, positive pressure ventilation, and intubation as deemed necessary by the anesthesiologist.

NEUROLOGIC COMPLICATIONS RELATED TO THE SPINAL CORD
Direct Spinal Cord or Nerve Root Injury

The spinal cord ends at L1 in approximately 80% of the adult population and at L2 in the remaining 20%.[13] Therefore, staying below the L2 spinous process when performing any neuraxial technique helps to avoid damage to the terminal portion of the cord (the conus medullaris). Using Tuffier's line, the imaginary line joining the 2 iliac crests, as a landmark for the L3-L4 interspace or L4 spinous process is common but unreliable.[37] Clinicians' identification of specific levels is more often erroneous.[38] Direct cord injury may still occur by needle injury, catheter injury, or intraneural local anesthetic injection.

It is not uncommon for patients to experience fleeting paresthesias to the lower extremities during neuraxial needle and/or catheter placements, and these are not associated with long-term neurologic sequelae[13] If symptoms persist during manipulation it is prudent to stop and reposition the needle and/or catheter. Long-term neurologic symptoms are rare but of concern, and will merit a neurology consultation with possible radiologic and nerve conduction studies.

Indirect Spinal Cord Injury

Epidural hematoma

Symptoms Epidural hematomas are a rare but devastating complication of neuraxial techniques. Their incidence is 1 in 200,000 with spinal techniques versus 1 in 150,000 with epidural techniques.[39] Despite the engorgement of epidural vessels during pregnancy, hematomas are a rare occurrence in the obstetric population,[38] with an incidence of 1 in 500,000 to 700,000 epidural procedures.[2,38] A recent study of electronic data sets from 11 academic centers reported no hematomas requiring laminectomy in a total of 79,837 epidural catheterizations in obstetric patients.[40] The decreased incidence compared with nonpregnant patients is thought to be due to relative hypercoagulability and a decreased likelihood of canal or foraminal stenoses (**Boxes 7–9**).

If a patient has risk factors for abnormal bleeding, laboratory studies such as platelet count and coagulation panel should be obtained before performing any neuraxial procedures. Thromboelastography has been characterized for pregnant patients, and has become an option, if available, to evaluate the patient's coagulation function.[41]

Diagnostic tests Diagnosis is made by consideration of patient risk factors and symptoms of new onset. A high index of suspicion should trigger neurosurgical consultation, and radiologic imaging with CT or MRI.

Treatment Treatment usually requires emergent surgical decompression, preferably within 6 hours from onset of symptoms, to avoid or minimize permanent neurologic deficits.[42–45]

Epidural abscess

Symptoms An infectious complication of epidural placement, an epidural abscess has catastrophic consequences. Its incidence in the obstetric population is reported to be approximately 1 in 500,000 epidural procedures.[2] Skin flora, specifically *Staphylococcus aureus,* is the most usual causative agent (**Box 10, Table 9**).[26,37]

Box 7
Symptoms of an epidural hematoma

- Epidural anesthesia persisting for more than the expected duration of the local anesthetic given
- Back pain
- Local back tenderness
- Persistent numbness and/or motor weakness of lower extremities
- Sphincter dysfunction

Box 8
Differential diagnosis of epidural hematoma

- Back soreness from epidural placement
- Back pain of other cause
- Epidural abscess
- Normal persistent motor block from local anesthetics
- Spinal infarction
- Spinal tumor
- Disc disease
- Nerve irritation from obstetric/delivery etiology

Box 9
Risk factors for epidural bleeding

- Gestational thrombocytopenia, idiopathic thrombocytopenic purpura
- Preeclampsia/eclampsia
- HELLP syndrome (hemolysis, elevated liver enzymes, and low platelets)
- Inherited clotting disorders
- Use of anticoagulant or antiplatelet agents
- Spinal deformity
- Traumatic needle and/or catheter placement
- Spinal tumor
- Clinical history of abnormal bleeding

Diagnosis and treatment Diagnosis is made by a constellation of clinical symptoms with laboratory tests consistent with infection. Confirmation is made by MRI. Treatment may be conservative, with antibiotics for 2 to 4 weeks, although most patients also require percutaneous drainage or laminectomy.[13,46–49]

Box 10
Differential diagnosis for epidural abscess

- Disc and degenerative bone disease
- Spinal tumor
- Vertebral discitis and osteomyelitis
- Meningitis
- Herpes zoster, before the appearance of skin lesions
- Epidural hematoma
- Spinal infarction
- Meningitis
- Multiple sclerosis

Table 9
Epidural abscess

Risk Factors	Symptomatology
Prolonged epidural catheter placement	Severe back pain with local tenderness
Poor aseptic technique during epidural placement equipment	Radiating dermatomal pain
	Headache
Multiple attempts at insertion	Malaise
Traumatic insertion	Fever
Patient with depressed immunity: steroids, diabetes mellitus, human immunodeficiency virus	Leg weakness
	Paresthesias
	Paraplegia
Body fluids in the bed	Bladder and bowel dysfunction
Preexisting maternal sepsis[2]	Elevated white blood cell count and C-reactive protein[26]
	Leaking of fluid at needle insertion site[26]

Vascular Injury

Anterior spinal artery syndrome

Symptoms Ischemic injury to the spinal cord is unusual in the obstetric population, in whom arterial disease is rare and hypotension is treated aggressively.[37] Blood supply to the anterior two-thirds of the spinal cord is provided by a single anterior spinal artery with reinforcement from radicular arteries originating from the thoracolumbar area.[50,51] If blood supply is compromised, anterior spinal artery syndrome occurs with loss of motor, pain, and temperature function below the level of the lesion. Bladder and bowel incontinence also is present (**Box 11**, **Tables 10** and **11**).

Box 11
Differential diagnosis of anterior spinal artery syndrome

- Arteriovenous malformations
- Atlantoaxial instability
- Compressive mass lesions/neoplasms
- Dissection syndromes
- Epidural hematoma
- Leptomeningeal carcinomatosis
- Metastatic disease to the spine and related structures
- Neurosarcoidosis
- Neurosyphilis
- Polyarteritis nodosa
- Spinal cord hemorrhage
- Syringomyelia
- Tuberculous meningitis
- Varicella zoster
- Vasculitis
- Viral meningitis

Data from Scott TF. Spinal cord infarction. Available at: http://emedicine.medscape.com/article/1164217-overview. Accessed February 3, 2013.

Table 10
Diagnostic approach for anterior spinal artery syndrome

Laboratory Workup[52]	Imaging/Others
CBC: leukocytosis suggests an infectious cause of spinal cord compromise	MRI
Fasting serum glucose: diabetes mellitus is a risk factor for epidural abscess and vascular disease	Electromyography and nerve conduction studies
ESR, ANA: autoimmune causes	
Lipid panel: vascular risk factor	
Serologic test for syphilis	
Electrolytes: potassium imbalances can be related to paresis	
CSF analysis: infectious and autoimmune causes	

Abbreviations: ANA, antinuclear antibodies; CBC, complete blood count; CSF, cerebrospinal fluid; ESR, erythrocyte sedimentation rate; MRI, magnetic resonance imaging.

Table 11
Therapy for acute spinal artery syndrome

Anticoagulation: aspirin vs antiplatelet agents	Consultations
Leg-compression devices	Neurosurgery
Low-dose subcutaneous heparin	Physiatry
	Neurorehabilitation

Chemical Injury

Cauda equina syndrome

Symptoms Cauda equina syndrome refers to a constellation of conditions whereby compression or irritation of the cauda equina nerve roots becomes symptomatic. After regional anesthesia, it results from neurotoxicity caused by local anesthetics in the intrathecal space. Historically it was first attributed to the use of continuous intrathecal microcatheters; however, lidocaine maldistribution or pooling in a small area, especially near the sacral roots, has been identified as the cause (**Boxes 12** and **13, Table 12**).[13]

Box 12
Differential diagnosis of cauda equina syndrome

- Disc herniation
- Lesions in other portions of the spinal cord
- Metastatic disease
- Multiple sclerosis
- Pernicious anemia
- Tabes dorsalis
- Tumors of the spinal cord (ependymoma, chordoma, meningioma)

Box 13
Diagnosis and treatment of cauda equina syndrome

Diagnosis

Imaging studies are the mainstay of diagnosis:

- MRI
- CT scan

Treatment[53,54]

Treatment is directed to the cause

- If inflammatory cause suspected: NSAIDs and steroids
- If infectious etiology suspected: Antibiotics
- Physical and occupational therapy consultation
- If due to mass effect: Surgical decompression surgery within 48 hours of onset

Table 12
Cauda equina syndrome

Risk Factors[1]	Symptomatology
Spinal block failure, followed by repeated injection	Burning low back pain
Fine-gauge or pencil-point needle	Sphincter dysfunction
Spinal microcatheters	Paraplegia
Continuous infusion	Sensory dysfunction in the perineum
Hyperbaric anesthetic solution	(saddle anesthesia)
Lithotomy position	
Intrathecal injection of a large volume intended for the epidural space	
Incorrect formulation, with unsuitable preservative or antioxidant	
Intrathecal lidocaine, particularly 5% (to a lesser degree, dibucaine, mepivacaine, and tetracaine)	

Transient neurologic syndrome/transient radicular irritation

Symptoms Transient neurologic syndrome (TNS) or transient radicular irritation (TRI) typically presents a day or two after spinal anesthesia. Back pain and radicular-like symptoms radiating to the buttocks or lower extremities are typical, without specific neurologic deficits. Risk factors are similar to those of anesthetic-induced cauda equina syndrome. As with cauda equina syndrome, irritation of the nerves by an intrathecal injection is the most likely cause.[26] Symptoms resolve on their own, usually in a few days, and are managed with NSAIDs. Parturients seem to be at a lower risk than other surgical patients,[26] and there is a higher incidence with the lithotomy position. The syndrome can be triggered by any anesthetic, but occurs most frequently with lidocaine and very rarely with bupivacaine.[37,55]

Diagnosis TNS/TRI is a clinical diagnosis. MRI, neurologic, and electrophysiologic examinations will be normal.

Treatment Although potentially causing distress to both the patient and health care provider, TNS is a benign, self-limited entity that requires only conservative therapy, and usually resolves without intervention within a few days.[56–58] Patient reassurance is key, and pharmacologic therapy with NSAIDs and opioids may be helpful.

Arachnoiditis

Symptoms Chronic adhesive arachnoiditis may cause long-term derangements via inflammation and scarring caused by a chemical injury to the pia-arachnoid.[59] These scars can impede CSF flow, disrupt blood supply, and cause atrophy.[4] Symptoms are delayed and include severe back pain that increases with activity, unilateral or bilateral leg pain, and an abnormal neurologic examination.[60] In extreme cases, paraplegia results. Some of the precipitating factors are contamination with:

1. Blood (in the setting of subarachnoid hemorrhage)
2. Local anesthetics (controversial)
3. Preservatives/antioxidants in local anesthetics
4. Contamination of local anesthetics with irritating chemicals
5. Detergents
6. Bactericidal cleansing agents: alcohol, chlorhexidine

Diagnosis Diagnosis of arachnoiditis is made by clinical presentation and radiologic imaging with CT or MRI. These radiologic methods have replaced myelograms, which require dyes that exacerbate symptoms.

The classic radiologic findings on MRI include short caudal sac appearance resulting from the adhesion of the nerve roots within the meninges, and irregular filling defects resulting from scar tissue (**Box 14**).[60,61]

Treatment There is no specific cure for arachnoiditis. Supportive management is focused on relieving pain that impairs daily activities. Methods of treatment include opioids, steroids, and spinal cord stimulation. Surgical removal of scar tissue is regarded as a last resort after conservative treatments have been exhausted.[61]

Back Pain

Nonspecific back pain after delivery is common and is similar in incidence (44%) whether or not epidural analgesia is used.[2,62] Previously controversial, studies show there is no causal relationship between neuraxial procedures and chronic low back pain.[2,62–64] A study of 369 women, published in the *British Medical Journal*, concluded: "After childbirth there are no difference in long-term low back pain, disability or movement restriction between women who receive epidural pain relief and women who receive other forms of pain relief."[63] However, transient tenderness at the site of the epidural needle insertion is common, and should resolve within a few days. Factors contributing to this localized tenderness include:

1. Multiple attempts
2. Traumatic manipulation
3. Ligamentous injury
4. Periosteal trauma
5. Local inflammation

Box 14
Differential diagnosis of arachnoiditis

- Spinal cord tumors
- Cauda equina syndrome
- Arachnoiditis ossificans
- Syringomelia
- Failed back syndrome

Box 15
Differential diagnosis of pregnancy-related back pain

- Urinary tract infection
- Osteomyelitis
- Lumbar disc lesion/prolapse
- Arthritis of spine/hip
- Lumbar stenosis
- Cauda equina syndrome
- Spondylolisthesis
- Pregnancy-associated osteoporosis
- Femoral vein thrombosis
- Osteitis pubis
- Rupture of symphysis pubis
- Sciatica
- Obstetric complications (preterm labor, abruption, red degeneration of uterine fibroid, round ligament pain, and chorioamnionitis)

Data from Vermani E, Mittal R, Weeks A. Pelvic girdle pain and low back pain in pregnancy: a review. Pain Pract 2010;10(1):60–71.

More generalized peripartum back pain can have multiple causes, including:

1. Hormonal changes causing ligamentous softening and joint laxity
2. Increased back lordosis caused by the mechanical changes of having an enlarged uterus
3. Increased mechanical load on joints with nerve root compromise

A comprehensive history and physical examination are needed to rule out more serious etiology of back pain.

Potential "red flags" include history of trauma, steroid use, unexplained weight loss, fever, and pain that does not improve with rest and is of disabling nature.[65] The presence of neurologic deficits such as bowel and bladder dysfunction requires emergent neurosurgical consultation. Although the diagnosis of pregnancy-related back pain is made clinically, imaging such as MRI may be necessary to rule out other serious causes of back pain (**Box 15**).

Management is based on a multidisciplinary approach, which includes[65]:

- Patient education
- Physical therapy and exercise
- Massage and heat therapy
- Transcutaneous electrical stimulation
- Acupuncture[66,67]
- Pharmacotherapy: NSAIDs, opioids

PERIPHERAL NERVE INJURY SECONDARY TO OBSTETRIC BIRTH TRAUMA
Introduction

Peripheral nerve injury related to birth trauma is common and is often erroneously attributed to neuraxial analgesia/anesthesia.[13] In 2 prospective studies, the incidence

Box 16
Risk factors for peripheral nerve injury

- Nulliparity
- Prolonged second stage of labor
- Cephalopelvic disproportion
- Nonvertex fetal presentation
- Forceps-assisted vaginal delivery
- Retractor use during cesarean delivery

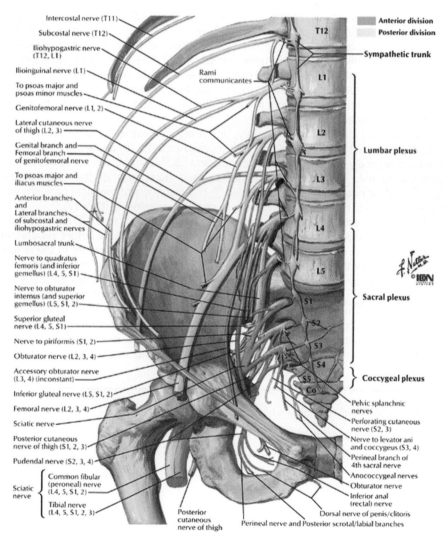

Fig. 1. Spinal nerve innervation. (Netter illustration from www.netterimages.com. © Elsevier Inc. All rights reserved.)

of obstetric palsies with a motor deficit was 24% and 37%.[68] Injury can be caused by direct compression or stretch of the nerve with impairment of the neurovascular supply (**Box 16, Fig. 1**).[2,68]

Neuraxial techniques can indirectly contribute to these neuropathies when there is failure to recognize symptoms of nerve injury or when a dense block allows a patient to remain for prolonged periods in positions that would otherwise be uncomfortable.[2,68] Prolonged second stage of labor with prolonged pushing in the lithotomy position can increase the risk of nerve injury.[2,68] Symptoms of obstetric nerve palsies are usually transient, with a mean duration of 6 to 8 weeks.

Presentation

The lumbosacral plexus is composed of the lumbar plexus (ventral rami of L1–L4 spinal nerves) and the sacral plexus (ventral rami of L5–S4 spinal nerves). It is most commonly injured by compression of the fetal head against the posterior rim of the pelvic bone or during instrumental vaginal delivery. Owing to its relationship to the bony pelvis, the common peroneal nerve component of the lumbosacral plexus is more commonly injured than the tibial component.[68] The injury may be unilateral (75%) or even bilateral (25%), and may involve multiple root levels.[13,62] Clinical manifestations of lumbosacral plexus injury include weakness of quadriceps and hip adductors, foot drop, numbness of the lateral lower leg and dorsum of the foot, and dysfunction of the anal sphincter.

Lateral femoral cutaneous nerve injury, or meralgia paresthetica, is the most common peripartum nerve injury.[2] This nerve is located superficially under the inguinal ligament and is purely sensory; derived from L2 and L3.[69] Compression or stretch injury manifests as mild discomfort, paresthesias, and numbness of the anterolateral thigh.[69–71] Most cases are unilateral (80%).[69] The diagnosis of meralgia paresthetica before childbirth is not a contraindication to regional anesthesia (**Box 17**).[71]

The common peroneal nerve originates from nerve roots L4 to S2.[72] It arises from the lateral side of the sciatic nerve and winds around the fibular neck before separating into superficial and deep branches.[64] The superficial branch is sensory to the lateral leg and dorsum of the foot while the deep part is motor to ankle and toe extensors. The nerve is particularly susceptible to injury because of its proximity to the bone and minimal superficial protection[2]; injury occurs via compression of the nerve against the fibular head. This injury may occur with pressure from leg braces and side rails, inappropriate positioning of the legs in stirrups, prolonged lithotomy or squatting, and even hand pressure on the lateral leg while the patient is pushing.[68,71,73–76] The nerve palsy can manifest with paresthesia in the lateral calf and dorsum of the foot,

---

Box 17
Risk factors for lateral femoral cutaneous nerve injury

- Prolonged pushing in the lithotomy or stirrups position (hip flexion)
- Increased abdominal pressure: obesity and pregnancy
- Diabetes
- Trauma
- Exaggerated lumbar lordosis
- Stretching or pressure by a retractor during cesarean delivery
- External pressure (by a belt or tight clothing)

foot drop, and inversion.[63,73] The femoral nerve is the largest branch of the lumbar plexus,[2] originating from nerve roots L2 to L4. At the turn of the twentieth century, postpartum femoral neuropathy was fairly common.[13] The use of active labor protocols has decreased injuries to the femoral nerve, although it remains the second most common intrinsic obstetric palsy.[13] The femoral nerve does not descend into the true pelvis, so compression injury occurs not with the fetal head[37,64] but rather along its anatomic path beneath the inguinal ligament on its way to the thigh. This compression is most likely to occur with prolonged labor, cephalopelvic disproportion, lithotomy position, or the use of retractor blades during a cesarean delivery.[77,78] Femoral nerve palsy may present with a patient falling when trying to get out of bed to ambulate, or with impaired ability to climb stairs.[2,63] Other typical findings include thigh and leg paresthesias, and an inability to flex at the hip or extend at the knee.[63] Femoral neuropathies have a good prognosis as long as the compression is relieved.[64] Demyelinating lesions usually recover completely within 3 to 4 months.[64]

The obturator nerve originates from nerve roots L2 to L4 and passes through the obturator canal on the lateral pelvic wall.[72] Descending into the true pelvis, its most common mechanism of injury is via compression between the pelvis and fetal head during childbirth, or compression by forceps applied to the fetal head.[13,38,64,72] Compression by hematomas, as a complication of pudendal nerve block, also leads to entrapment of the nerve.[13] Nerve injury manifests with numbness of the medial thigh and abnormal gait secondary to weakness of thigh adductors.[79,80] Adductor weakness can be masked by femoral and sciatic nerve compensation. Functional recovery is typically good; however, chronic pain syndromes may occur with severe injury (**Table 13**).[64]

Table 13 Peripheral nerve innervation			
Nerve	**Nerve Root**	**Sensory Loss**	**Motor Loss**
Lumbosacral plexus	L4–S5	Lateral calf Lateral foot	Hip extension Hip abduction Foot flexion
Lateral femoral cutaneous	L2, L3	Anterolateral thigh	None
Common peroneal	L4–S2	Anterolateral leg and dorsum of foot and toes	Foot dorsiflexion and eversion
Femoral	L2, L3, L4 (anterior)	Anteromedial thigh Medial calf Medial foot	Hip flexion Knee extension Patellar reflex
Obturator	L2, L3, L4 (posterior)	Medial thigh Medial knee	Thigh adduction

Data from Tsen LC. Neurologic complications of labor analgesia and anesthesia. Int Anesthesiol Clin 2002;40(4):67–88.

Diagnosis and Management

A focused and comprehensive history and physical examination are crucial to the diagnosis of peripheral nerve injuries (**Table 14**).

If symptoms worsen, neurologic consultation is warranted, and other studies might be indicated:

- MRI
- CT scan
- Electroencephalogram

Table 14
Diagnostic approach to pregnancy-related peripheral nerve injury

History[13]

Onset

Location and severity

Progression or regression

Neuraxial anesthesia: paresthesias during procedure, location, recovery from neuraxial anesthesia

Duration of labor: position, duration of pushing, instrumentation (vacuum, forceps)

Physical Examination[69]			
Root/Muscle	**Motor**	**Sensory**	**Reflexes**
L1–2 Iliopsoas	Hip flexion	Groin, anterior thigh	
L3 Abductor longus, brevis, manus, minimus	Hip adduction	Anterior knee, anterior lower leg	Knee jerk
L3–4 Quadriceps femoris	Knee extension		Knee jerk
L4 Tibialis anterior	Knee extension	Medial lower leg and ankle	Knee jerk
L5 Extensor halluces longus, brevis Extensor digitorum longus, brevis Gluteus medius	Toe extension Hip abduction	Anterolateral lower leg and dorsum of foot	Hamstring jerk
L5–S1 Semitendinosus Semimembranosus Biceps femoris	Knee flexion		
S1 Gastrocnemius Soleus Flexor digiti brevis	Ankle flexion Foot eversion Toe flexion	Sole and lateral border foot and ankle	Ankle jerk

- Electromyogram
- Nerve conduction studies

Symptoms of birth trauma–related neuropathies improve or resolve in almost all patients; the median duration of symptoms is 6 to 8 weeks. Based on the duration, it is likely that the cause of the injuries is minor degrees of axon loss or focal demyelination.[81,82] Conservative therapy such as minimizing periods of standing, eliminating tight clothing, and using oral analgesics may facilitate recovery.[71] Effective communication with the patient, family members, and primary obstetric team is key for addressing the patient's concerns, implementing support measures for the patient, and ensuring appropriate follow-up.

SUMMARY

Neuraxial anesthesia has significantly enhanced the experience of childbirth, revolutionized the management of labor pain and has decreased maternal morbidity and mortality. Nonetheless, a wide range of neurologic issues can arise secondary to neuraxial anesthesia as well as the birth process. Some of the most common neurologic complaints that will come to the attention of anesthesiologists include headaches and peripheral nerve injuries. While serious complications are rare, even minor complications are problematic to patients who are otherwise healthy and for whom uninterrupted time with newborns is valued. Even though anesthetic procedures can cause neurologic sequelae, these are much less frequent than those caused by birth trauma.

REFERENCES

1. Macarthur A. Chapter 31. Postpartum headache. In: Chesnut DH, editor. Chestnut's obstetric anesthesia principles and practice. 4th edition. Philadelphia: Mosby Elsevier; 2009. p. 677–700.
2. Chang LY, Carabuena JM, Camann W. Neurologic issues and obstetric anesthesia. Semin Neurol 2011;31(4):374–84.
3. Sprigge JS, Harper SJ. Accidental dural puncture and post dural puncture headache in obstetric anaesthesia: presentation and management: a 23-year survey in a district general hospital. Anaesthesia 2008;63(1):36–43.
4. Bradbury CL, Singh SI, Badder SR, et al. Prevention of post-dural puncture headache in parturient: a systematic review and meta-analysis. Acta Anaesthesiol Scand 2013;57:417–30.
5. Gaiser R. Postdural puncture headache. Curr Opin Anaesthesiol 2006;19: 249–53.
6. Baysinger CL, Pope JE, Lockhart EM, et al. The management of accidental dural puncture and postdural puncture headache: a North American survey. J Clin Anesth 2011;23(5):349–60.
7. Gaiser RR. Postdural puncture headache: a headache for the patient and a headache for the anesthesiologist. Curr Opin Anaesthesiol 2013;26(3):296–303.
8. Ghaleb A. Review article: postdural puncture headache. Anesthesiol Res Pract 2010. http://dx.doi.org/10.1155/2010/102967.
9. Ho KY, Gan TJ. Management of persistent post-dural puncture headache after repeated epidural blood patch. Acta Anaesthesiol Scand 2007;51(5):633–6.
10. Collier BB. Treatment for post dural puncture headache. Br J Anaesth 1994; 72(3):366–7.
11. Fry RA, Perera A. Failure of repeated blood patch in the treatment of spinal headache. Anaesthesia 1989;44:492–3.
12. Nepomuceno R, Herd A. Bilateral subdural hematoma after inadvertent dural puncture during epidural analgesia. J Emerg Med 2012;44(2):e227–30.
13. Kowe O, Waters JH. Neurologic complications in the patient receiving obstetric anesthesia. Neurol Clin 2012;30(3):823–33.
14. Delfyett WT, Fetzer DT. Imaging of neurologic conditions during pregnancy and the perinatal period. Neurol Clin 2012;30(3):791–822.
15. Wagner AL. Imaging in subdural hematoma. Available at: http://emedicine.medscape.com/article/344482-overview. Accessed January 20, 2013.
16. Zeidan A, Farhat O, Maaliki H, et al. Does postdural puncture headache left untreated lead to subdural hematoma? Case report and review of the literature. Middle East J Anesthesiol 2010;20(4):483–92.
17. Kayacan N, Arici G, Karsli B, et al. Acute subdural haematoma after accidental dural puncture during epidural anaesthesia. Int J Obstet Anesth 2004;13(1):47–9.
18. Kim YD, Lee JH, Cheong YK. Pneumocephalus in a patient with no cerebrospinal fluid leakage after lumbar epidural block—a case report. Korean J Pain 2012;25(4):262–6.
19. Smarkusky L, DeCarvalho H, Bermudez A, et al. Acute onset headache complicating labor epidural caused by intrapartum pneumocephalus. Obstet Gynecol 2006;108(3 Pt 2):795–8.
20. Schirmer CM, Heilman CB, Bhardwaj A. Pneumocephalus: case illustrations and review. Neurocrit Care 2010;13(1):152–8.
21. Dexter F, Reasoner DK. Theoretical assessment of normobaric oxygen therapy to treat pneumocephalus. Anesthesiology 1996;84(2):442–7.

22. Gore PA, Maan H, Chang S, et al. Normobaric oxygen therapy strategies in the treatment of postcraniotomy pneumocephalus. J Neurosurg 2008;108(5): 926–9.
23. Lee LC, Lieu FK, Chen YH, et al. Tension pneumocephalus as a complication of hyperbaric oxygen therapy in a patient with chronic traumatic brain injury. Am J Phys Med Rehabil 2012;91(6):528–32.
24. Lee CH, Chen WC, Wu CI, et al. Tension pneumocephalus: a rare complication after hyperbaric oxygen therapy. Am J Emerg Med 2009;27(2):257.
25. Gómez-Ríos MÁ, Fernández-Goti MC. Pneumocephalus after inadvertent dural puncture during epidural anesthesia. Anesthesiology 2013;118(2):444.
26. Reynolds F. Neurological infections after neuraxial anesthesia. Anesthesiol Clin 2008;26(1):23–52. http://dx.doi.org/10.1016/j.anclin.2007.11.006, v.
27. Baer ET. Post-dural puncture bacterial meningitis. Anesthesiology 2006;105(2): 381–93.
28. Mhyre JM. What's new in obstetric anesthesia in 2009? An update on maternal patient safety. Anesth Analg 2010;111(6):1480–7.
29. Lewis G. Saving mothers' lives: reviewing maternal deaths to make motherhood safer, 2003-2005. London: CEMACH; 2007.
30. Spence AG. Lipid reversal of central nervous system symptoms of bupivacaine toxicity. Anesthesiology 2007;107:516–7.
31. Toledo P. The role of lipid emulsion during advanced cardiac life support for local anesthetic toxicity. Int J Obstet Anesth 2011;20(1):60–3.
32. Toledo P, Nixon HC, Mhyre JM, et al. Brief report: availability of lipid emulsion in United States obstetric units. Anesth Analg 2013;116(2):406–8.
33. Hiller DB, Gregorio GD, Ripper R, et al. Epinephrine impairs lipid resuscitation from bupivacaine overdose: a threshold effect. Anesthesiology 2009;111: 498–505.
34. Mulroy MF. Systemic toxicity and cardiotoxicity from local anesthetics: incidence and preventive measures. Reg Anesth Pain Med 2002;27(6):556–61.
35. Lofsky AS. Doctors Company reviews maternal arrests cases. APSF Newslett 2007;22:28.
36. Davies JM, Posner KL, Lee LA, et al. Liability associated with obstetric anesthesia: a closed claims analysis. Anesthesiology 2009;110:131–9.
37. Bader A. Chapter 32. Neurologic complications of pregnancy and neuraxial anesthesia. In: Chesnut DH, editor. Chestnut's obstetric anesthesia principles and practice. 4th edition. Philadelphia: Mosby Elsevier; 2009. p. 701–26.
38. Hogan Q. Epidural catheter tip position and distribution of injectate evaluated by computed tomography. Anesthesiology 1999;90(4):964–70.
39. Brooks H, May A. Neurological complications following regional anesthesia in obstetrics. Br J Anaesth 2003;3:111–4.
40. Bateman BT, Mhyre JM, Ehrenfeld J, et al. The risk and outcomes of epidural hematomas after perioperative and obstetric epidural catheterization: a report from the multicenter perioperative outcomes group research consortium. Anesth Analg 2013;116(6):1380–5.
41. Karlsson O, Sporrong T, Hillarp A, et al. Prospective longitudinal study of thromboelastography and standard hemostatic laboratory tests in healthy women during normal pregnancy. Anesth Analg 2012;115(4):890–8.
42. Guffey PJ, McKay WR, McKay RE. Case report: epidural hematoma nine days after removal of a labor epidural catheter. Anesth Analg 2010;111(4): 992–5.
43. Pear BL. Spinal epidural hematoma. Am J Roentgenol 1972;115:155–64.

44. Badar F, Kirmani S, Rashid M, et al. Spontaneous spinal epidural hematoma during pregnancy: a rare obstetric emergency. Emerg Radiol 2011;18(5): 433–6.
45. Ruppen W, Derry S, McQuay H, et al. Incidence of epidural hematoma, infection, and neurologic injury in obstetric patients with epidural analgesia/anesthesia. Anesthesiology 2006;105(2):394–9.
46. Grewal S, Hocking G, Wildsmith JA. Epidural abscesses. Br J Anaesth 2006; 96(3):292–302.
47. Chiang HL, Chia YY, Chen YS, et al. Epidural abscess in an obstetric patient with patient-controlled epidural analgesia—a case report. Int J Obstet Anesth 2005; 14(3):242–5.
48. Green LK, Paech MJ. Obstetric epidural catheter-related infections at a major teaching hospital: a retrospective case series. Int J Obstet Anesth 2010;19(1): 38–43.
49. Evans PR, Misra U. Poor outcome following epidural abscess complicating epidural analgesia for labour. Eur J Obstet Gynecol Reprod Biol 2003;109(1):102–5.
50. Eastwood DW. Anterior spinal artery syndrome after epidural anesthesia in a pregnant diabetic patient with scleroderma. Anesth Analg 1991;73:90–1.
51. Zuber WF, Gaspar MR, Rothschild PD. The anterior spinal artery syndrome—a complication of abdominal aortic surgery: report of five cases and review of the literature. Ann Surg 1970;172(5):909–15.
52. Scott TF. Spinal cord infarction. Available at: http://emedicine.medscape.com/ article/1164217-overview. Accessed February 3, 2013.
53. Shivji F, Tsegaye M. Cauda equina syndrome: the importance of complete multidisciplinary team management. BMJ Case Rep 2013.
54. Chabbouh T, Lentschener C, Zuber M, et al. Persistent cauda equina syndrome with no identifiable facilitating condition after an uneventful single spinal administration of 0.5% hyperbaric bupivacaine. Anesth Analg 2005;101(6):1847–8.
55. Freedman JM, Li DK, Drasner K, et al. Transient neurologic symptoms after spinal anesthesia: an epidemiologic study of 1,863 patients. Anesthesiology 1998; 89(3):633–41.
56. Harned ME, Dority J, Hatton KW. Transient neurologic syndrome: a benign but confusing clinical problem. Adv Emerg Nurs J 2011;33(3):232–6.
57. Zaric D, Pace NL. Transient neurologic symptoms (TNS) following spinal anaesthesia with lidocaine versus other local anaesthetics. Cochrane Database Syst Rev 2009;(2):CD003006.
58. Liberman A, Karussis D, Ben-Hur T, et al. Natural course and pathogenesis of transient focal neurologic symptoms during pregnancy. Arch Neurol 2008; 65(2):218–20.
59. Killeen T, Kamat A, Walsh D, et al. Severe adhesive arachnoiditis resulting in progressive paraplegia following obstetric spinal anaesthesia: a case report and review. Anaesthesia 2012;67(12):1386–94.
60. Rice I, Wee MY, Thomson K. Obstetric epidurals and chronic adhesive arachnoiditis. Br J Anaesth 2004;92(1):109–20.
61. Wright MH, Denney LC. A comprehensive review of spinal arachnoiditis. Orthop Nurs 2003;22(3):215–9.
62. Zawkowski M. Obstetric related neurologic complications. Soap Winter Newsletter 2012:6–2.
63. Macarthur AJ, Macarthur C, Weeks SK. Is epidural anesthesia in labor associated with chronic low back pain? A prospective cohort study. Anesth Analg 1997;85(5):1066–70.

64. Howell CJ, Dean T, Lucking L, et al. Randomised study of long term outcome after epidural versus non-epidural analgesia during labour. BMJ 2002; 325(7360):357.
65. Vermani E, Mittal R, Weeks A. Pelvic girdle pain and low back pain in pregnancy: a review. Pain Pract 2010;10(1):60–71.
66. Furlan AD, van Tulder M, Cherkin D, et al. Acupuncture and dry-needling for low back pain: an updated systematic review within the framework of the Cochrane Collaboration. Spine (Phila Pa 1976) 2005;30(8):944–63.
67. Ee CC, Manheimer E, Pirotta MV, et al. Acupuncture for pelvic and back pain in pregnancy: a systematic review. Am J Obstet Gynecol 2008;198(3):254–9.
68. Wong CA. Nerve injuries after neuraxial anaesthesia and their medicolegal implications. Best Pract Res Clin Obstet Gynaecol 2010;24(3):367–81.
69. Tsen LC. Neurologic complications of labor analgesia and anesthesia. Int Anesthesiol Clin 2002;40(4):67–88.
70. Bradshaw AD, Advincula AP. Postoperative neuropathy in gynecologic surgery. Obstet Gynecol Clin North Am 2010;37(3):451–9.
71. Van Diver T, Camann W. Meralgia paresthetica in the parturient. Int J Obstet Anesth 1995;4(2):109–12.
72. Russel DR, Reynolds F. Long term backache after childbirth: prospective search for causative factors. BMJ 1996;312(7043):1384–8.
73. Chung KH, Lee JY, Ko TK, et al. Meralgia paresthetica affecting parturient women who underwent cesarean section—a case report. Korean J Anesthesiol 2010;59(Suppl):S86–9.
74. Radawski MM, Strakowski JA, Johnson EW. Acute common peroneal neuropathy due to hand positioning in normal labor and delivery. Obstet Gynecol 2011; 118(2 Pt 2):421–3.
75. Qublan HS, al-Sayegh H. Intrapartum common peroneal nerve compression resulted in foot drop: a case report. J Obstet Gynaecol Res 2000;26(1):13–5.
76. Babayev M, Bodack MP, Creatura C. Common peroneal neuropathy secondary to squatting during childbirth. Obstet Gynecol 1998;91(5 Pt 2):830–2.
77. Cohen S, Zada Y. Postpartum femoral neuropathy. Anaesthesia 2001;56(5): 500–1.
78. Kofler M, Kronenberg MF. Bilateral femoral neuropathy during pregnancy. Muscle Nerve 1998;21(8):1106.
79. Nogajski JH, Shnier RC, Zagami AS. Postpartum obturator neuropathy. Neurology 2004;63(12):2450–1.
80. Hong BY, Ko YJ, Kim HW, et al. Intrapartum obturator neuropathy diagnosed after cesarean delivery. Arch Gynecol Obstet 2010;282(3):349–50.
81. Wong CA, Scavone BM, Dugan S, et al. Incidence of postpartum lumbosacral spine and lower extremity nerve injuries. Obstet Gynecol 2003;101(2):279–88.
82. Sahai-Srivastava S, Amezcua L. Compressive neuropathies complicating normal childbirth: case report and literature review. Birth 2007;34(2):173–5.

Effects of General Anesthesia During Pregnancy on the Child's Ability to Learn

Tammy Euliano, MD

KEYWORDS

- Developmental neurotoxicity • Cell death • Anesthesia
- Apoptotic neurodegeneration

KEY POINTS

- Substantial animal data suggest anesthetics cause long-lasting histologic and behavioral effects.
- Effects depend on dose and timing of the exposure relative to the brain growth spurt.
- Retrospective studies in children exposed to surgery/anesthesia as infants demonstrate an association with learning disabilities, especially with multiple exposures.
- Twin studies show no such association.
- Fetal effects in humans have not been documented, but studies are limited.
- Ongoing studies are aggressively seeking to determine whether this risk is real and how to minimize the impact of necessary surgery and anesthesia prenatally and on young children.

About 2% of pregnant women will require surgery before delivery. The possibility that maternal exposure to anesthetics impact the child's future cognitive function was recognized almost 40 years ago. Quimby and colleagues[1] investigated the effect of trace environmental anesthetic gases on cognition, perception, and motor reaction. One of the exposure groups was pregnant rats; their pups demonstrated "enduring deficits in learning tasks,"[1] as well as evidence of neuronal degeneration and failure of synapse formation. With adult-only exposure, however, no functional deficit and minimal neuronal damage was detected. Additional studies followed, to minimal fanfare, mostly in rats and with prolonged exposures, multiple confounders, and end points of questionable clinical significance.

In 1999, the issue reached the lay press via *Science* with Ikonomidou and colleagues'[2] report that N-methyl-d-aspartate (NMDA)–receptor antagonists caused neuronal loss in rats, the location and degree of which depended on the timing of

Department of Anesthesiology, University of Florida College of Medicine, Box 100254, 1600 Southwest Archer Road, Gainesville, FL 23610, USA
E-mail address: teuliano@ufl.edu

Anesthesiology Clin 31 (2013) 595–607
http://dx.doi.org/10.1016/j.anclin.2013.04.003
1932-2275/13/$ – see front matter © 2013 Elsevier Inc. All rights reserved.

exposure in late fetal and early neonatal life. Within 2 years, that article had been cited 66 times and was followed by a series of rat studies by Jevtovic-Todorovic's[3] group demonstrating not only neurodegeneration but also persistent learning deficits. Soon the pediatric anesthesia world was awash with parental questions and frequent articles on the potential long-term effects of anesthetic exposure early in childhood.[4] Although the need for surgery persists, evidence for the safest anesthetic remains elusive.

FETAL BRAIN DEVELOPMENT

As a multistep process, the development of the nervous system is, not surprisingly, highly complex. Beginning with the formation of the neural tube, neuroblasts appear in abundance via mitosis. The excess (30%–50%) eventually undergoes apoptosis, programmed cell death. The survivors migrate and grow axons and dendrites. Following the development of electrical polarity, the critical phase of synaptogenesis ensues.[5] The initial overly exuberant synapse formation requires pruning, an activity-dependent process that depends on calcium channels. Active neurons seek out one another while their listless cousins in effect implode.[6] Adverse effects of anesthetics on this process have been identified at several stages, primarily dendrite formation and synaptogenesis, together with presumably unintended apoptosis.

Although all mammals have similar developmental stages, the timings vary considerably (**Fig. 1**). The vulnerable brain growth spurt in humans is thought to extend from

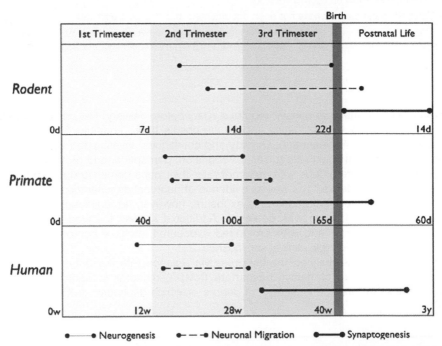

Fig. 1. Comparison of major fetal neurodevelopmental events across mammalian species. Diagrammatic collation of multiple studies to simplify understanding of the timelines of major neurodevelopmental events in utero. Events are as marked in the legends (d, days; w, weeks; y, years). Synaptogenesis is predominantly a postnatal event in rodents, unlike primates and humans. (*From* Palanisamy A. Maternal anesthesia and fetal neurodevelopment. Int J Obstet Anesth 2012;21:152–62; with permission.)

at least the third trimester (and possibly earlier) through 2 to 4 years of age. This period is narrower in primates and only days long in the much-studied rodents. The period of peak synaptogenesis in the human varies with the area of the brain, proceeding from the sensorimotor cortex in utero to the prefrontal cortex by 3 years of age. For interference with synaptogenesis to play a role in anesthesia-induced neurodevelopmental impairment, susceptibility should mirror these phases; experimental design should include tests specific for the brain area under development at the time of the exposure. For example, exposure at 2 years of age would likely affect executive function (ie, the ability to plan, make decisions, and make good choices socially, as parents frequently cajole).

MOLECULAR EFFECTS OF ANESTHESIA ON BRAIN DEVELOPMENT

Prenatal ethanol exposure has been the target of much research.[7] Its influence on brain development is multifaceted, depending on the dose and timing; at least some mechanisms overlap with those of volatile agents. In particular, the inhibition of NMDA-glutamate receptors and activation of gamma-aminobutyric acid (GABA) receptors cause the upregulation of caspase-3, an executioner protease that begins the cascade of apoptotic cell death (see later discussion).

In the immature brain, the normally inhibitory neurotransmitter (GABA) is excitatory. In fact, it is the principal excitatory transmitter stimulating synapse formation, modulating migration of new neurons to their target sites.[8] Anesthetic antagonism of GABA-receptors presents a clear opportunity for neurodevelopmental effects.

Neuroapoptosis

Apoptosis (from Greek for "falling off") is also termed programmed cell death or cellular suicide. Unlike cells that die of acute injury or hypoxia, which typically swell and burst (necrosis), the less familiar and less dramatic apoptotic cell death occurs from the inside, without affecting neighboring cells. The cell basically disintegrates and helpfully arranges for its own removal by displaying cell surface proteins easily recognized by macrophages.[9] The details of the apoptotic process are still being worked out, and there are likely several pathways (**Fig. 2**). In simple terms, an internal or external trigger results in a cascade ending with the dismantling of the cellular structure.[10] Anesthetic agents can trigger this pathway through at least 3 proposed pathways (see **Fig. 2**).[11]

Additional potential mechanisms include the inhibition of the formation of mature brain-derived neurotrophic factor from its precursor in the synapse; buildup of the precursor stimulates apoptosis and inhibits synaptogenesis. Isoflurane and sevoflurane may both increase the amount and activity of β-amyloid (implicated in Alzheimer's disease) leading to apoptosis.[12] Finally, neuroinflammation may be a common pathway of cognitive impairment and offers avenues for therapeutic research.[13]

EVIDENCE IN NEONATAL ANIMALS

Early investigations into the anesthetic effects on the developing brain used neonatal rodents and conclusively demonstrated detrimental effects on synapse formation and remodeling, neuronal cytoskeleton formation, and glial cell growth and maturation.[14] Altered performance on various neurobehavioral tasks is also undisputed, but the relationship between the two remains conjecture. Major criticisms of the animal studies included the rodents' very brief brain growth phase (2 weeks), relatively high doses of anesthetics (although minimum alveolar concentration [MAC] in rodents is higher than that in humans), extensive duration of anesthetic relative to life span

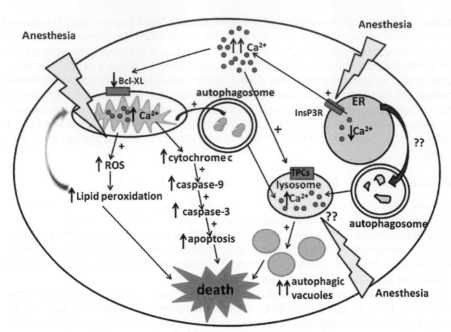

Fig. 2. Anesthesia-induced pathways of developmental neurodegeneration. Three pro-posed pathways are focused on mitochondria, endoplasmic reticuli (ER), and lysosomes: (1) ER-dependent pathway involves anesthesia-induced activation of inositol 1,4,5-trisphos-phate receptors (InsP3R) leading to the excessive calcium (Ca^{2+}) release and acute elevation of cytosolic Ca^{2+}. This change causes downregulation of mitochondrial anti-apoptotic pro-tein, Bcl-XL, which in turn induces cytochrome c leak in the cytoplasm. Cytochrome c acti-vates the mitochondrial apoptotic pathway by activating caspase-9 and -3 leading to DNA fragmentation and neuronal death. (2) Mitochondria-dependent pathway also involves anesthesia-induced upregulation of reactive oxygen species (ROS) leading to the excessive lipid peroxidation of lipid membranes and damage to neuronal organelles, mitochondria, and ER in particular. Because damaged mitochondria become an uncontrollable source of ROS and cytochrome c, and damaged ER become an uncontrollable source of cytosolic Ca^{2+}, they have to be removed by autophagy leading to the excessive formation of auto-phagosomes and increase in autophagic load. (3) The lysosome-dependent pathway in-volves lysosome activation via nicotinic acid adenine dinucleotide phosphate (NAADP)–gated 2-pore channels (TPCs), which control Ca^{2+} uptake into the lysosomes. An increase in the intralysosomal level of Ca^{2+} activates lysosomal activity, which in turn promotes lyso-somal and autophagosomal fusion, the formation of autophagic vacuoles, and neuronal self-eating. Although it is proposed that anesthesia causes lysosomal activation indirectly via an increase in cytosolic Ca^{2+} from the ER, it remains unclear whether anesthesia has a direct effect on lysosomal activation (via NAADP-gated TPCs in particular). (*From* Jevtovic-Todorovic V, Boscolo A, Sanchez V, et al. Anesthesia-induced developmental neurodegener-ation: the role of neuronal organelles. Front Neurol 2013;3:1–7; with permission.)

(eg, 4–6 hours in a 2-year lifespan), the inability to adequately monitor their cardiopul-monary system during exposure, and, of course, the fact they are rodents.

However, studies in nonhuman primate newborns have shown similar results with evidence of neuroapoptosis[15] and glial cell death[16] with as little as 5 hours of isoflur-ane exposure at a clinically relevant concentration. Others have found that a combina-tion of agents (eg, isoflurane plus nitrous oxide) is required for neuronal damage.[17]

Behaviorally, 24 hours of ketamine at a "light surgical plane"[18] during the first week of life significantly disrupted performance in tests of neurocognitive function even 3.5 years later.[18]

IN UTERO ANIMAL STUDIES

Less prevalent are studies of in utero anesthetic exposure, but these show similar results. Palanisamy and colleagues[19] exposed pregnant rats at midgestation to 4 hours of 1.4% isoflurane ($\sim$1 MAC). The offspring were studied in adulthood (8 weeks of age) with various tasks and found to have impaired spatial memory acquisition. They did eventually learn but more slowly than the controls.

Similarly, Zheng and colleagues[20] found that the progeny of midgestation pregnant mice exposed to just 2 hours of 2.5% sevoflurane suffered learning and memory impairment in adulthood (31 days). In this study, the investigators also showed increases in markers of neuroinflammation and neuronal damage in the sevoflurane-exposed group. Perhaps more interesting, environmental enrichment (social interaction and novel stimulation for 2 hours per day beginning antepartum and continuing with mom and pups together throughout the study period) reversed the sevoflurane-induced changes, rescuing the system from neuroinflammation and synaptic loss and improving learning and memory.

Guinea pigs' brain growth spurt is 5 times the duration of that in rodents and much of it occurs prenatally. Rizzi and colleagues[21] found that anesthetic exposure during pregnancy causes significant severe and widespread apoptosis leading to fewer neurons in key areas of the brain. The severity of effect was proportional to the number of agents to which the guinea pigs were exposed: isoflurane alone, isoflurane plus midazolam, isoflurane plus nitrous oxide, or all 3. However, no neurobehavioral testing was performed for clinical correlation in this study.

A substantial criticism in all of these animal studies is the lack of a surgical intervention. In fact, the addition of noxious stimulation in rat pups, concurrent with 6 hours of ketamine exposure, *attenuated* the neuroapoptotic response to ketamine alone.[22]

HUMAN STUDIES

The compelling evidence in animals begged for human studies, yet ethical considerations have hampered progress. There are numerous barriers to this research:

- There is a lack of an appropriate control group: surgery without anesthesia is inhumane, and anesthesia without surgery is unethical.
- There is a poorly defined brain growth spurt period in humans (for determining the specific vulnerable period).
- There is a lack of a well-defined and consensus outcome. A diagnosis of learning disability (LD) may vary with local definitions; school performance has numerous confounders. For prospective studies, the selected test battery must be practicable and specific for the anticipated neurobehavioral effects, which vary with timing and dose of exposure.
- There are numerous known confounders: gender, parental educational attainment, socioeconomic status, environment, overall health and need for surgery, birth and childhood events, and so forth.
- There are unknown confounders: perhaps dietary, medication or environmental exposures, and likely many others.

- There is an extensive lag period for results. The neurobehavioral effects of an anesthetic performed during gestation or early childhood cannot be evaluated for years. Many patients will be lost to follow-up.

Recognizing these barriers, initial studies have been retrospective in nature (**Table 1**). Ing and colleagues[23] appropriated data previously acquired to investigate the impact of prenatal ultrasound in Australia. After removal of those patients lost to follow-up, the dataset included 1781 children of which 258 were exposed to anesthesia before 3 years of age (52 with multiple exposures), according to parental diaries (no medical records were available). Several times through 10 years of age, the patients underwent a battery of tests to assess language, cognitive function, motor skills, and behavior. Unlike most other studies, this group found a demonstrable difference in performance on receptive/expressive language even with a single exposure (adjusted risk ratios of 1.73–2.41 depending on the test); the effect increased with multiple exposures. No differences were found in behavior or motor function. The thoroughness of the testing is a strength of this study and provides an opportunity to detect subtle effects. There are, however, several weaknesses. The inclusion criteria were perhaps too broad; nearly 15% of the procedures were circumcision or "minor skin and nail procedures,"[23] for which there may have been no anesthesia provided. Also included were patients having cardiac and neurosurgical procedures, a major confounder for neurologic outcomes.

Olmsted County Dataset

A group at Rochester's Mayo Clinic has performed multiple related analyses using a rich data set: children born between 1976 and 1982 in Olmsted County, Minnesota. Data include birth details, childhood anesthetic/surgical records, and school/standardized test performance as well as results of evaluations for LD. The investigators defined LD using standard local formulae based on IQ and standardized test performance. Excluding those patients with severe mental retardation (n = 19) and the 6% whose parents declined participation resulted in a cohort of 5357 patients.

Of the 5357 patients, 593 (11%) underwent a procedure requiring general anesthesia before 4 years of age. Using a multivariate analysis to control for confounders in the anesthesia-exposed children (lower birth weight, lower gestational age, and fewer girls), the investigators found that a single anesthetic exposure (n = 449) was not associated with an increased incidence of LD. However, multiple exposures and a longer cumulative duration of anesthesia did increase the risk. The hazard ratio (HR) with more than 2 exposures was 2.60 (95% confidence interval [CI] 1.60, 4.24).[24] Because children requiring multiple operations likely suffer additional confounders of chronic disease, the investigators separately analyzed only those patients with an American Society of Anesthesiology Physical Class of less than 3 with the same result.

The investigators acknowledged that this association does not prove causation, and there are numerous other limitations. Once a child met the criteria for LD, they remained in that cohort. Because the definition was based on the expected standardized test outcome relative to IQ, a poor day on a standardized test or an erroneously high IQ score would both cause possible mislabeling of an otherwise normally functioning child. With regard to the patients, this area of Minnesota at the time was not representative of the United States, with few minorities in the cohort. Also, patients were followed only until they were diagnosed with LD, died, or moved out of the area. The investigators assumed, with some previous data to back them up, that the portion of the cohort that emigrated did not differ from those studied. They did not report the number of patients whose academic records were available through

Table 1
Human neonatal studies on neurodevelopmental effects

Author	Population	Target Group	Exposure Timing	Sample vs Control Group Size	Outcome	Hazard or Odds Ratio
Ing et al,[23] 2012	Western Australia Pregnancy Cohort	Any anesthetic exposure	<3 y	258 vs 1781	Language, cognitive function, motor skills, and behavior through 10 y of age	Language: 2.68 for multiple, 2.36 for single
Sprung et al,[26] 2012	Olmsted	Any anesthetic exposure	<2 y	341 vs 5016	ADHD by 19 y of age	None for single, 1.95 for >1 operations
Wilder et al,[24] 2009	Olmsted	Any anesthetic exposure	<4 y	593 vs 4764	LD diagnosis	None for single, 1.59 for 2 operations, 2.60 for >2 operations
Flick et al,[25] 2011	Olmsted	Any anesthetic exposure	<2 y	350 vs 700, matched	LD diagnosis	None for single, 2.12 for >1 operations
DiMaggio et al,[27] 2009	NY Medicaid	Inguinal hernia repair	<3 y	383 vs 5000	Developmental or behavioral disorder	2.3
Hansen et al,[28] 2011	Danish hospital register	Hernia repair	<1 y	2689 vs 14 575	Ninth grade test scores and teacher ratings	None
DiMaggio et al,[30] 2011	NY Medicaid	Multiple exposures	<3 y	304 vs 10 146	Developmental or behavioral disorder	None for single, 2.9 for 2 operations, 4.0 for >2 operations
Twin Studies						
Bartels et al,[29] 2009	Netherlands Twin Register	Any anesthetic exposure	<3 y	130 discordant vs 948 concordant pairs	Standardized test and teacher rating of cognitive skills at 12 y of age	None
DiMaggio et al,[30] 2011	NY Medicaid	Multiple exposures	<3 y	138 discordant twin pairs	Developmental or behavioral disorder	None

Abbreviations: ADHD, attention-deficit/hyperactivity disorder; LD, learning disability.

19 years of age, thus there could be many more LD-labeled children from either group. With regard to the extrapolation to current practice, most of the anesthetics administered were halothane/nitrous oxide, rarely used today.

Narrowing the cohort slightly, another study focused on patients exposed to anesthesia before 2 years of age.[25] These patients were matched to unexposed controls based on the identified risk factors for LDs, including gender, mother's education, birth weight, gestational age, and current patient age. Those with repeated (but not single) exposure had an increased risk of developing LD (HR 2.12, 95% CI 1.26, 3.54) but not the need for Individualized Educational Programs (IEPs) related to emotional or behavioral disorders.

Conversely, another study on the same data sample identified a nearly doubled risk of being diagnosed with attention-deficit/hyperactivity disorder (ADHD) in those exposed to multiple (HR 1.95; 95% CI 1.03, 3.71) but not single (HR 1.18; 95% CI 0.79, 1.77) procedures requiring general anesthesia.[26] The apparent discrepancy between the studies is attributed to a different endpoint: patients can have an ADHD diagnosis without requiring an IEP.

Inguinal Hernia Repair Studies

Inguinal hernia repair is a common operation in infancy, usually performed using a brief general anesthetic, thus providing a viable dataset for investigating neurocognitive outcomes.

Using a retrospective cohort analysis of a New York Medicaid database, DiMaggio and colleagues[27] compared 383 children who underwent inguinal hernia surgery before 3 years of age with more than 5000 controls matched by age but having no history of hernia repair. Notably, there was no effort to eliminate controls that had non-hernia surgery before 3 years of age, and they did not attempt to determine the type of anesthetic used. Those who underwent hernia surgery had more than double the risk of being diagnosed with a developmental or behavioral disorder, even after controlling for age, gender, and birth-related complications (adjusted HR 2.3, 95% CI 1.3, 4.1). In fact, what this study showed is that Medicaid patients who require hernia repair early in childhood have more developmental problems later. It cannot distinguish whether factors associated with the development of the hernia itself (eg, prolonged mechanical ventilation as a neonate), the hernia operation, or the anesthesia in particular are to blame.

Meanwhile, a similar study found no such association. Using Danish hospital records, Hansen and colleagues[28] reviewed the academic performance of all children born between 1986 and 1990 who underwent hernia repair in infancy (<1 year, n = 2689) with an age-matched random 5% population sample (n = 14,575). The investigators used scores on a ninth grade national standardized test and average teacher rating as their academic performance metric. After controlling for confounders (gender, birth weight, parental age, and education), there was no difference between the infants who had hernia repair and the control group. However, there was a small increase in test nonattainment in the former group. This increase in nonattainment "most often denotes children with special needs that prohibit them from following the standard ninth grade course curriculum"[28] but also includes dropouts and children who choose alternative schools. The continuous academic performance metric used in this study differs substantially from the binary outcome (LD diagnosis) used in other studies, complicating comparison. Similar to the DiMaggio study discussed earlier,[27] the investigators did not confirm that patients in the control group had no nonhernia-related anesthetic exposures, and the limitation of the surgical group to the first year of life is much stricter than the DiMaggio cohort.

On balance, the data to this point suggest that early surgery in childhood, and especially multiple operations, may have an effect on future performance, even after controlling for some obvious confounders. But other likely significant variables remain.

Twin Studies

Bartels and colleagues[29] hypothesized that the need for surgery and the genetic background for that need affects cognitive performance rather than the anesthetic exposure. They used the Netherlands Twin Register to identify monozygotic twins born between 1986 and 1995. After eliminating twins with severe handicap, born before 32 weeks or with a birth weight less than 2000 g, the investigators reviewed 1143 pairs. Results of nationwide intermittent parental surveys were used to determine anesthetic exposure before 3 years of age and between 3 and 12 years of age. Educational achievement was measured by standardized test performance at 12 years of age. Similar to other studies, children exposed to anesthesia before 3 years of age had lower achievement scores and more cognitive problems; however, when looking only at discordant twins pairs (whereby one was exposed and the other not), there was no difference. Twins tended to perform like each other regardless of anesthetic exposure, and those twins who both received anesthesia did underperform relative to pairs whereby neither was anesthetized. The investigators site this as evidence that the underlying nature/nurture that necessitates surgery correlates with educational performance rather than the surgery/anesthesia itself. Limitations of this study include lack of information regarding type, duration, and number of anesthetics as well as the use of parental recall and survey return for data collection. Further, there is no mention of the age at which individual students took the eighth grade examination. A student who repeated a year in school might have an LD not detected by an examination taken after additional schooling.

DiMaggio and colleagues[30] found similar results using the New York State Medicaid database. Although the 304 children exposed to anesthesia more than once before 3 years of age were more likely to be diagnosed with a developmental or behavioral disorder than the 10,146 unexposed children (2.9, 95% CI 2.5, 3.1), and this risk increased with the number of surgeries (≥ 3 4.0, 95% CI 3.5, 4.5), there was no increased risk in matched analysis of 138 sibling pairs.

These last two studies, although far from conclusive, provide welcome reassurance. However, much of human neurodevelopment occurs prenatally.

IN UTERO HUMAN STUDIES

In a small study (n = 29), women who underwent appendectomy during pregnancy were surveyed regarding their child's subsequent motor, sensory, and social development. No developmental delays were identified by 3 years of age, regardless of the trimester in which the surgery occurred.[31]

The Olmsted County dataset described earlier was used to investigate a relationship between learning disabilities and the type of anesthesia administered for cesarean delivery.[32] Of the 497 patients born by cesarean, nearly 40% underwent general anesthesia. Although high by today's standards, this was the national average at the time.[33] Children born using maternal general or regional anesthesia for cesarean delivery were not more likely to develop LDs than their vaginally delivered counterparts. In fact, the subgroup born by cesarean using regional anesthesia had the lowest incidence of LD (HR 0.64, 95% CI 0.44, 0.92 relative to vaginal delivery).

This last finding prompted the group to hypothesize that the stress of labor might affect neurobehavioral outcomes and that neuraxial analgesia for vaginal delivery might be protective. They found no such association in the same cohort of patients.[34]

PLANNED OUTCOME STUDIES

In 2008, the International Anesthesia Research Society and the Food and Drug Administration joined forces in SmartTots (Strategies for Mitigating Anesthesia-Related neuroToxicity in Tots), an advisory group of experts from academia and industry whose mission is to direct and fund research in this area. Their scientific advisory board has developed a research agenda beginning with additional animal studies and progressing through translation to nonhuman primates.[35]

There are at least 2 major ongoing studies: (1) The General Anesthesia Study compares awake spinal with sevoflurane general anesthesia for inguinal herniorraphy.[36] The primary outcome of this study is the IQ at 5 years of age, but they will also examine additional neurodevelopmental and behavioral outcomes. (2) The Pediatric Anesthesia NeuroDevelopment Assessment (PANDA) project uses an ambidirectional design. After identifying sibling pairs discordant for inguinal hernia repair before 36 months of age, the investigators are prospectively performing several neuropsychological assessments. A pilot feasibility study of 28 sibling pairs has helped refine the protocol and demonstrated its feasibility.[37]

NEUROPROTECTIVE STRATEGIES?

Before effective preventive strategies are studied, the proof that anesthetics have detrimental neurodevelopmental effects, the mechanism of these effects, and the anesthetic options and potential treatments to prevent the undesirable side effects must be established. However, the treatment must not introduce new problems (eg, prevent apoptosis, including the normal apoptosis required for development). In the meantime, finding preventative agents helps elucidate causes:

- Lithium counteracts a precursor step (phosphorylation of extracellular signal-regulated protein kinase) in ethanol-induced neuroapoptosis. This step is also important for the neuroapoptotic actions of ketamine and propofol, which are prevented with lithium coadministration.[38]
- Upregulation of reactive oxygen species causes lipid peroxidation and mitochondrial damage (see **Fig. 2**). Agents that scavenge reactive oxygen species or restore mitochondrial integrity prevent anesthesia-induced cognitive impairment,[39] including melatonin[40] and 1.3% hydrogen gas.[41]
- L-type calcium channel blockers may inhibit excessive calcium influx, which leads to apoptosis.[42] Similarly, an increase in calcium binding proteins, as may be induced by vitamin D_3, is protective.[43]
- Alpha-2 agonists have neuroprotective properties and activate survival pathways. Clonidine abolishes ketamine's adverse effects on apoptosis and behavior in mice,[44] whereas dexmedetomidine attenuates the isoflurane-induced effects on long-term memory in rats, an effect that is reversed by the blockade of α_2 but not GABA receptors.[45] A similar activation of prosurvival proteins may explain the neuroprotective effects of 17β-estradiol.[46]
- Nonsteroidal anti-inflammatory medications (eg, ketorolac) inhibit the proinflammatory cytokines that induce neurobehavioral deficits in sevoflurane.[13]
- Hypothermia prevents both natural and anesthesia-induced neuroapoptosis in mice.[47]

- Preconditioning may reduce adverse effects as it does with ischemia. Both small doses of ketamine and xenon may be neuroprotective by this mechanism.[43]
- Environmental enrichment several weeks after sevoflurane exposure in rats[48] and in the perioperative period for mice[20] reversed the deleterious effects on short-term memory and other tests of cognitive function.

SUMMARY

Incriminating data are extensive in the neonatal animal literature, with somewhat less in utero data available. The studies in humans are less extensive and a bit less compelling. Meanwhile, the twin studies provide hope.[29,30] Although most studies found children who undergo surgery early in childhood (particularly those who require multiple operations) underperform their healthy counterparts, those differences evaporate when controlling for the maximum possible confounders. Ongoing studies seek to provide additional answers as to the effects, mechanisms, and prevention strategies as well as suggest the optimal anesthetic for pregnant women and neonates.

REFERENCES

1. Quimby KL, Aschkena LJ, Bowman RE, et al. Enduring learning deficits and cerebral synaptic malformation from exposure to 10 parts of halothane per million. Science 1974;185:625–7.
2. Ikonomidou C, Bosch F, Miksa M, et al. Blockade of NMDA receptors and apoptotic neurodegeneration in the developing brain. Science 1999;283:70–4.
3. Jevtovic-Todorovic V, Hartman RE, Izumi Y, et al. Early exposure to common anesthetic agents causes widespread neurodegeneration in the developing rat brain and persistent learning deficits. J Neurosci 2003;23:876–82.
4. Davidson A, Soriano S. Does anaesthesia harm the developing brain - evidence or speculation? Paediatr Anaesth 2004;14:199–200.
5. Sarnat HB, Flores-Sarnat L. Developmental disorders of the nervous system. In: Daroff RB, Fenichel GM, Jankovic J, et al, editors. Bradley's neurology in clinical practice. Philadelphia: Elsevier Saunders; 2012. p. 1396–421.
6. Stoneham ET, Sanders EM, Sanyal M, et al. Rules of engagement: factors that regulate activity-dependent synaptic plasticity during neural network development. Biol Bull 2010;219:81–99.
7. Alfonso-Loeches S, Guerri C. Molecular and behavioral aspects of the actions of alcohol on the adult and developing brain. Crit Rev Clin Lab Sci 2011;48:19–47.
8. Ben Ari Y, Gaiarsa JL, Tyzio R, et al. GABA: a pioneer transmitter that excites immature neurons and generates primitive oscillations. Physiol Rev 2007;87: 1215–84.
9. Alberts B, Johnson A, Lewis J, et al. Programmed cell death (apoptosis). Molecular biology of the cell. New York: Garland Science; 2002.
10. Blaylock M, Engelhardt T, Bissonnette B. Fundamentals of neuronal apoptosis relevant to pediatric anesthesia. Paediatr Anaesth 2010;20:383–95.
11. Jevtovic-Todorovic V, Boscolo A, Sanchez V, et al. Anesthesia-induced developmental neurodegeneration: the role of neuronal organelles. Front Neurol 2013;3: 1–7.
12. Vlisides P, Xie ZC. Neurotoxicity of general anesthetics: an update. Curr Pharm Des 2012;18:6232–40.
13. Shen X, Dong YL, Xu ZP, et al. Selective anesthesia-induced neuroinflammation in developing mouse brain and cognitive impairment. Anesthesiology 2013;118: 502–15.

14. Jevtovic-Todorovic V. Anesthesia and the developing brain: are we getting closer to understanding the truth? Curr Opin Anaesthesiol 2011;24:395–9.
15. Brambrink AM, Evers AS, Avidan MS, et al. Isoflurane-induced neuroapoptosis in the neonatal rhesus macaque brain. Anesthesiology 2010;112:834–41.
16. Brambrink AM, Back SA, Riddle A, et al. Isoflurane-induced apoptosis of oligodendrocytes in the neonatal primate brain. Ann Neurol 2012;72:525–35.
17. Zou XJ, Liu F, Zhang X, et al. Inhalation anesthetic-induced neuronal damage in the developing rhesus monkey. Neurotoxicol Teratol 2011;33:592–7.
18. Paule MG, Li M, Allen RR, et al. Ketamine anesthesia during the first week of life can cause long-lasting cognitive deficits in rhesus monkeys. Neurotoxicol Teratol 2011;33:220–30.
19. Palanisamy A, Baxter MG, Keel PK, et al. Rats exposed to isoflurane in utero during early gestation are behaviorally abnormal as adults. Anesthesiology 2011;114:521–8.
20. Zheng H, Dong YL, Xu ZP, et al. Sevoflurane anesthesia in pregnant mice induces neurotoxicity in fetal and offspring mice. Anesthesiology 2013;118:516–26.
21. Rizzi S, Carter LB, Ori C, et al. Clinical anesthesia causes permanent damage to the fetal guinea pig brain. Brain Pathol 2008;18:198–210.
22. Liu JR, Liu Q, Li J, et al. Noxious stimulation attenuates ketamine-induced neuroapoptosis in the developing rat brain. Anesthesiology 2012;117:64–71.
23. Ing C, DiMaggio C, Whitehouse A, et al. Long-term differences in language and cognitive function after childhood exposure to anesthesia. Pediatrics 2012;130:E476–85.
24. Wilder RT, Flick RP, Sprung J, et al. Early exposure to anesthesia and learning disabilities in a population-based birth cohort. Anesthesiology 2009;110:796–804.
25. Flick RP, Katusic SK, Colligan RC, et al. Cognitive and behavioral outcomes after early exposure to anesthesia and surgery. Pediatrics 2011;128:E1053–61.
26. Sprung J, Flick RP, Katusic SK, et al. Attention-deficit/hyperactivity disorder after early exposure to procedures requiring general anesthesia. Mayo Clin Proc 2012;87:120–9.
27. DiMaggio C, Sun LS, Kakavouli A, et al. A retrospective cohort study of the association of anesthesia and hernia repair surgery with behavioral and developmental disorders in young children. J Neurosurg Anesthesiol 2009;21:286–91.
28. Hansen TG, Pedersen JK, Henneberg SW, et al. Academic performance in adolescence after inguinal hernia repair in infancy a nationwide cohort study. Anesthesiology 2011;114:1076–85.
29. Bartels M, Althoff RR, Boomsma DI. Anesthesia and cognitive performance in children: no evidence for a causal relationship. Twin Res Hum Genet 2009;12:246–53.
30. DiMaggio C, Sun LN, Li GH. Early childhood exposure to anesthesia and risk of developmental and behavioral disorders in a sibling birth cohort. Anesth Analg 2011;113:1143–51.
31. Choi JJ, Mustafa R, Lynn ET, et al. Appendectomy during pregnancy: follow-up of progeny. J Am Coll Surg 2011;213:627–32.
32. Sprung J, Flick RP, Wilder RT, et al. Anesthesia for cesarean delivery and learning disabilities in a population-based birth cohort. Anesthesiology 2009;111:302–10.
33. Gibbs CP, Krischer J, Peckham BM, et al. Obstetric anesthesia - a national survey. Anesthesiology 1986;65:298–306.
34. Flick RP, Lee K, Hofer RE, et al. Neuraxial labor analgesia for vaginal delivery and its effects on childhood learning disabilities. Anesth Analg 2011;112:1424–31.

35. Ramsay JG, Rappaport BA. SmartTots: a multidisciplinary effort to determine anesthetic safety in young children. Anesth Analg 2011;113:963–4.
36. Davidson AJ, Mccann ME, Morton NS, et al. Anesthesia and outcome after neonatal surgery the role for randomized trials. Anesthesiology 2008;109:941–4.
37. Sun LS, Li GH, DiMaggio CJ, et al. Feasibility and Pilot Study of the Pediatric Anesthesia NeuroDevelopment Assessment (PANDA) project. J Neurosurg Anesthesiol 2012;24:382–8.
38. Straiko MM, Young C, Cattano D, et al. Lithium protects against anesthesia-induced developmental neuroapoptosis. Anesthesiology 2009;110:862–8.
39. Boscolo A, Starr JA, Sanchez V, et al. The abolishment of anesthesia-induced cognitive impairment by timely protection of mitochondria in the developing rat brain: the importance of free oxygen radicals and mitochondrial integrity. Neurobiol Dis 2012;45:1031–41.
40. Yon JH, Carter LB, Reiter RJ, et al. Melatonin reduces the severity of anesthesia-induced apoptotic neurodegeneration in the developing rat brain. Neurobiol Dis 2006;21:522–30.
41. Yonamine R, Satoh Y, Kodama M, et al. Coadministration of hydrogen gas as part of the carrier gas mixture suppresses neuronal apoptosis and subsequent behavioral deficits caused by neonatal exposure to sevoflurane in mice. Anesthesiology 2013;118:105–13.
42. Wei HF. The role of calcium dysregulation in anesthetic-mediated neurotoxicity. Anesth Analg 2011;113:972–4.
43. Turner CP, Gutierrez S, Liu C, et al. Strategies to defeat ketamine-induced neonatal brain injury. Neuroscience 2012;210:384–92.
44. Ponten E, Viberg H, Gordh T, et al. Clonidine abolishes the adverse effects on apoptosis and behaviour after neonatal ketamine exposure in mice. Acta Anaesthesiol Scand 2012;56:1058–65.
45. Sanders RD, Xu J, Shu Y, et al. Dexmedetomidine attenuates isoflurane-induced neurocognitive impairment in neonatal rats. Anesthesiology 2009;110:1077–85.
46. Asimiadou S, Bittigau P, Felderhoff-Mueser U, et al. Protection with estradiol in developmental models of apoptotic neurodegeneration. Ann Neurol 2005;58:266–76.
47. Creeley CE, Olney JW. The young: neuroapoptosis induced by anesthetics and what to do about it. Anesth Analg 2010;110:442–8.
48. Shih J, May LD, Gonzalez HE, et al. Delayed environmental enrichment reverses sevoflurane-induced memory impairment in rats. Anesthesiology 2012;116:586–602.

Amniotic Fluid Embolism

John M. Kissko III, MD*, Robert Gaiser, MD, MSEd

KEYWORDS

- Amniotic fluid embolism • Right heart failure • Transesophageal echocardiography
- Disseminated intravascular coagulopathy

KEY POINTS

- Amniotic fluid embolism (AFE) is a rare event, with an incidence of approximately 1 in 50,000 deliveries.
- AFE is typically a diagnosis of exclusion for a patient with sudden onset of hypotension followed by a coagulopathy. There are current blood tests that are highly specific and sensitive, but not commercially available.
- AFE tends to be a 2-step process of right heart failure followed by a coagulopathy. The leading theory is that it is an anaphylactoid reaction.
- There is no known treatment for AFE. The current therapy is supportive, addressing the hemodynamic effects and the coagulopathy.
- Outcomes following AFE remain with a mortality of 40% to 60%. The outcome for the neonate is also poor.

INTRODUCTION

Historically, an amniotic fluid embolism (AFE) was believed to be caused by an embolus of amniotic fluid into the maternal circulation from small tears in the uterus or cervix during or immediately after delivery, causing a physical obstruction of the pulmonary vasculature leading to sudden cardiovascular collapse. This belief was based on postmortem findings. First described in a 1926 case report, AFE was not assuredly defined until 1941, when Steiner and Lushbaugh[1] described postmortem examinations of patients who had suffered unexplained obstetric deaths, all with the same clinical picture. These autopsies showed pathology thought to be caused by amniotic fluid that had embolized to the pulmonary vasculature, including fat-positive aggregates and squamous epithelial cells. However, more recent studies have shown the presence of fetal squamous epithelial cells in the pulmonary arteries of women without any signs or symptoms of AFE[2]; current opinion is that AFE is a clinical syndrome, with the diagnosis depending on the clinical presentation rather than histopathologic findings.[3]

Department of Anesthesiology and Critical Care, University of Pennsylvania, 3400 Spruce Street, Philadelphia, PA 19104, USA
* Corresponding author.
E-mail address: john.kissko@uphs.upenn.edu

Anesthesiology Clin 31 (2013) 609–621
http://dx.doi.org/10.1016/j.anclin.2013.03.005
1932-2275/13/$ – see front matter
anesthesiology.theclinics.com

AFE is an extremely rare event that usually presents in the peripartum period (usually 30 minutes before to 30 minutes after delivery) although it has reportedly manifested at various times throughout pregnancy, and may occur as late as 48 hours postpartum.[3] Approximately 70% of cases occur before delivery; AFE also has been reported during or after induced abortion, intrapartum amnioinfusion, transabdominal amniocentesis, blunt abdominal trauma, surgical trauma, removal of cerclage, and manual removal of the placenta.[3] When AFE manifests after delivery, it has been suggested that amniotic fluid and fetal debris becomes trapped in the uterine veins at delivery, then released later into the circulation with uterine involution.[4]

The incidence of AFE is estimated to be between 1 in 8000 and 1 in 80,000 deliveries, depending on study definition.[5] According to the most recent analyses, the incidence of AFE ranges from 1 in 12,953 deliveries in the United States[6] to 1 in 56,500 in the United Kingdom.[7] Pooled data indicate an incidence in North America of 1 in 15,200[6,8,9] and in Europe, 1 in 53,800 deliveries.[7,10,11] These data represent all reported fatal and nonfatal cases of AFE, making the incidence likely even higher owing to underreporting, especially of nonfatal cases. An overall incidence is very difficult to estimate, secondary to poor reporting and a lack of a unifying definition of AFE.

The risk factors for AFE are not well established, primarily because there is no universal definition and the incidence is so low (**Box 1**). However, studies examining patients with acute hypotension, acute hypoxia, and coagulopathy, which occur during labor or within 30 minutes of delivery of the neonate without other clinical explanation, have documented certain commonalities that could be considered risk factors for AFE. Uterine hyperstimulation, specifically in the setting of augmented labor with the use of oxytocin, advanced maternal age, multiparity, cesarean delivery, placenta previa, placental abruption, cervical lacerations, instrumented vaginal delivery, eclampsia, uterine rupture, and male neonate are all reported risk factors for AFE.[6,9] Of note, maternal age less than 20 years and dystocia have been shown in epidemiologic studies to be protective against AFE. In these same studies, advanced maternal age in first pregnancy, primigravidity, high parity, previous cesarean sections, diabetes, multiple gestations, premature rupture of membranes, chorioamnionitis, and fetal macrosomia all had no influence on the incidence of AFE.

Box 1
Risk factors for amniotic fluid embolism

Uterine hyperstimulation

Use of oxytocin

Advanced maternal age

Multiparity

Cesarean delivery

Placenta previa

Placenta abruption

Cervical lacerations

Instrumented vaginal delivery

Eclampsia

Uterine rupture

Male neonate

Pathophysiology

Rather than an embolism of amniotic fluid causing physical obstruction of the pulmonary vasculature, AFE may better be described as an anaphylactoid reaction of pregnancy. There is usually no physical evidence of a clot burden causing pulmonary vascular obstruction. The clinical course of AFE is highly variable, with investigators being unable to consistently reproduce the effects of pulmonary vascular obstruction with amniotic fluid in animal models.[3] There have been several other suggested pathogenic mechanisms for AFE. Immunologic factors, complement and granulocyte activation by the amniotic fluid itself, and anaphylaxis secondary to one of many possible mediators in amniotic fluid (although these same investigators were then unable to demonstrate mast cell degranulation) have all been posited.[12–15]

The most likely pathophysiology of AFE is the entry of amniotic fluid into the maternal circulation with the resultant release of biochemical mediators, such as platelet-activating factor, histamine, bradykinin, endothelin, leukotrienes, or other arachidonic acid metabolites.[3] One or more of these mediators may lead to increased vascular permeability, bronchoconstriction, platelet aggregation, leukotriene, thromboxane and cytokine recruitment, and prostaglandin cascade (**Fig. 1**).

The exact mechanism of the coagulopathy in AFE is unknown. Laboratory experiments have shown that amniotic fluid decreases the clotting time of whole blood, induces platelet aggregation, produces a thromboplastin-like effect, and activates the complement cascade.[16] Tissue factor, which is present in amniotic fluid, also activates the extrinsic pathway by binding with factor VII and activating factor X, leading to clotting and the development of a consumptive coagulopathy.[17] A theory that

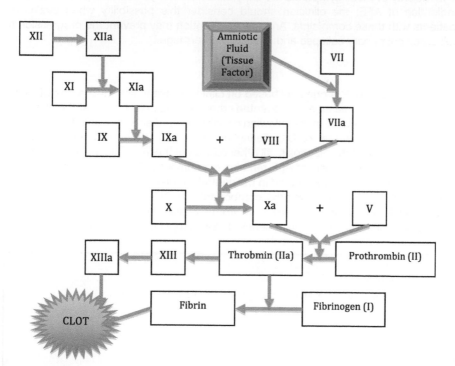

Fig. 1. Coagulation cascade: the role of amniotic fluid. Amniotic fluid, which contains tissue factor, has a role in the activation of the coagulation cascade by activating factor VII in the extrinsic pathway.

incorporates both the pulmonary and hematologic effects is this activation of the clotting cascade leading to microemboli in the pulmonary vasculature, which results in pulmonary vasoconstriction and the cardiovascular collapse.[18] Another group of investigators has also suggested that the disseminated intravascular coagulopathy (DIC) in AFE may actually be a result of complement activation rather than procoagulants entering the maternal circulation, when they found that all 8 of the women in their study who had experienced an AFE had abnormally low C3 and C4 complement levels.[14] Some investigators are questioning whether the majority of the bleeding seen in AFE is due to massive fibrinolysis rather than a consumptive coagulopathy. Two studies[19,20] have found evidence to the contrary, and the current consensus is that the hemorrhage seen in AFE is a result of DIC.

SYMPTOMS

The classic triad of AFE is sudden cardiovascular collapse, dyspnea, and DIC. According to the national AFE registry in the United States,[21] profound hypotension and fetal distress occurred in 100% of cases while cardiopulmonary arrest, pulmonary edema/acute respiratory distress syndrome, cyanosis, and coagulopathy occurred in 80% to 93%. Other less common signs and symptoms include nausea and vomiting, chest pain, dyspnea, paresthesias, agitation, or an "impending sense of doom." These signs and symptoms occur in varying degrees at various times (in combination or separately), and may wax and wane as AFE progresses. Symptoms may also occur immediately before cardiovascular collapse or reportedly as early as 4 hours prior.[22] The majority of these symptoms are early indicators of hypoxia, and provide an early indication of AFE; the clinician should consider this possibility when evaluating patients with these complaints. An early intervention may prevent the progression to full cardiopulmonary collapse and massive hemorrhage.

DIAGNOSIS

The diagnosis of AFE is primarily based on clinical presentation, and is one of exclusion. Roberts and colleagues[23] presented criteria for the diagnosis of AFE that include the presence of at least 1 of the following conditions: cardiac arrest, shock, severe respiratory distress, seizure, or DIC during pregnancy or within 48 hours of delivery (**Box 2**). To arrive at the diagnosis, all other causes of these events must be excluded.

The laboratory diagnosis of AFE remains experimental. The aspiration of amniotic fluid debris from a catheter located in the central circulation was thought to be pathognomonic for AFE. The histologic components of AFE that have been identified include: epithelial squamous cells shed from the skin, lanugo hair, vernix caseosa, mucin, and bile pigments.[24] In a series of 22 autopsies in women with presumed

---

Box 2
Diagnosis of AFE

The presence of at least 1 of the following within 48 hours of delivery:

Cardiac arrest

Shock

Severe respiratory distress

Seizure

Disseminated intravascular coagulopathy

AFE, only 16 (73%) had fetal elements identified in the pulmonary vasculature.[25] In cases where a distal port of the pulmonary artery catheter was aspirated, only 4 of the 8 cases had fetal elements in the aspirate. To add to the confusion, squamous cells have been identified in patients without AFE. In 5 patients with a pulmonary artery catheter and no evidence of AFE, blood samples were obtained. In 3 of the 5 samples of blood, squamous cells or lanugo hair were recovered, and in all of the samples, mucin was present.[25] Given the lack of specificity for the presence of these materials, other diagnostic criteria are helpful.

The clinical manifestations of AFE suggest it may be due to an anaphylactoid reaction.[3] Tryptase, a serine protease with a half-life of several hours, is released by mast cells. Tryptase is a serine protease that constitutes 20% of total mast cell protein. This protein has proved useful in the diagnosis of anaphylaxis or anaphylactoid reactions. A tryptase level greater than 1 ng/mL is considered elevated. Marcus and colleagues[26] presented a case of a parturient who had confirmed AFE by gross and microscopic findings and who also had a serum tryptase level of 11.4 ng/mL. However, a series of 9 patients with presumed AFE did not demonstrate elevated serum tryptase levels in any of the cases.[15] Given these results, serum tryptase levels have a very poor sensitivity.

The complement system helps the immune system remove pathogens. An alternative proposal for the pathophysiology of AFE is activation of the complement pathway. This theory is supported by studies measuring complement levels (C3 and C4). Of the 9 patients with presumed AFE, complement levels were severely depressed in comparison with those in postpartum controls.[15] The problem with complement activation is that it is nonspecific and may be decreased in patients with other disease states. In patients with clinical symptoms suggestive of AFE, decreased serum levels of C3 and C4 have sensitivities between 80% and 100% and a specificity of 100% for AFE.[15]

Zinc coproporphyrin 1 is present in amniotic fluid, and the elevation of the concentration of this protein in patients with AFE has been described. This compound is an attractive option as a possible biochemical marker of AFE, as coproporphyrins are found in meconium and the formation of a complex with zinc results in a fluorescent compound. The sera from 89 women were sampled for the presence of this compound. Of these samples, 4 were obtained from women with AFE as diagnosed by autopsy. The plasma concentration was greater than 35 nmol/L in the patients with AFE. Using this cutoff, the positive and negative predictive values and the specificity and sensitivity of prediction of AFE are 80%, 100%, 98%, and 100%, respectively.[27]

A more promising diagnostic test is measurement of insulin-like growth factor binding protein 1 (IGFBP1). This protein is a specific protein marker of amniotic fluid. In a series of 45 patients (25 with AFE and 20 without), IGFBP1 was higher in the serum of women with AFE than in those without. Parturients with AFE were identified when the patient had hypotension with 1 of the following signs with no clear cause: acute fetal compromise, cardiac arrest, cardiac rhythm problems, premonitory symptoms, seizure, shortness of breath, coagulopathy, maternal hemorrhage, and/or finding fetal squamous cells or hair in the lungs on postmortem examination. The non-AFE group had hypotension related to other causes. This biomarker has a high concentration in amniotic fluid, hence the increase with AFE. It is a protein primarily produced in the deciduas, and does not depend on fetal production. Using a cutoff concentration of greater than 87.5 μg/L, the test was 100% sensitive but 86.8% specific. Increasing the cutoff to greater than 104.5 μg/L decreased the sensitivity to 92% but increased the specificity to 97.8%.[28]

The laboratory diagnosis for AFE remains speculative. Tests that are easily obtainable, such as tryptase and complement, are nonspecific. The more diagnostic tests are purely experimental. It should be noted that the laboratory tests for zinc coproporphyrin 1 and IGFBP1 are not commercially available.

Transesophageal Echocardiography

The first case report describing the use of transesophageal echocardiography (TEE)[29] in the diagnosis of AFE is from 1999, in a term patient who presented at 40 weeks gestation for evaluation of vaginal bleeding. She was hemodynamically stable and asymptomatic at the time of admission, and her cervical examination was closed with 60% effacement. Oxytocin was used to augment her labor; within 80 minutes of starting the infusion, the patient started to complain of sudden-onset dyspnea, blindness, and palpitations. With subsequent maternal hypotension and persistent fetal bradycardia, the decision was made to perform an emergent cesarean delivery. The baby was delivered within 2 minutes of arriving at the operating room while cardiopulmonary resuscitation was being administered because of acute maternal cardiovascular collapse. A TEE probe was inserted, and the findings, which have been consistently demonstrated in several case reports since, indicated right heart failure with relatively preserved left heart function.

On long-axis 4-chamber view there was evidence of right ventricular failure, suprasystemic right-sided pressures, bulging of the interatrial and interventricular septae from right to left, severe tricuspid regurgitation, and a small pericardial effusion. The pulmonary artery systolic pressure was estimated at 45 mm Hg with no concurrent palpable arterial pulse. Of note, the left ventricle was small and compressed but appeared to have normal thickening and contraction laterally. The left ventricular septal wall, however, was not contracting normally and was in fact bulging significantly into the left ventricle, indicating right ventricular overload.

Before the publication of this case report, only a small number of human studies had looked at hemodynamic variables within the first hour of a recognized AFE, leading to the hypothesis that left heart failure with increased capillary wedge pressure leading to pulmonary edema was the primary cause of the cardiovascular collapse.[30–33] However, most studies implicating left heart failure as the major hemodynamic alteration associated with AFE were looking at patients who were 1 hour or more into the clinical syndrome.[3] This case report (the first using TEE in the diagnosis of AFE and the first to analyze AFE in its hyperacute stage) demonstrated involvement of the right heart, suggesting it as the first stage of an AFE response. This patient arrived at the operating room with no signs of left heart failure or pulmonary edema (normal oxygenation and lungs clear to auscultation). These investigators then theorized that AFE is a 2-stage response, with left heart failure and pulmonary edema only manifesting in those patients who survive the initial stage of right heart failure.

Several articles have looked at the use of TEE for the diagnosis of AFE since the publication of this landmark case report,[34,35] all of which have replicated the TEE findings in AFE: significant pressure and volume overload of the right heart altering the normal relationship between left and right ventricle, leading to the development of the classic D-shaped ventricle secondary to the altered dynamics of the interventricular septum. Other confirmatory signs of embolism, including an underloaded but normally contracting left ventricle, massively dilated pulmonary vasculature, and the lack of other cardiac abnormalities such as regional wall-motion abnormalities, valvular rupture or defects, intracardiac air, ventricular septal or atrial septal defects, or dynamic outflow obstruction, have also been demonstrated in subsequent case reports.

These case reports all appear to support the idea that the hemodynamic collapse seen in AFE is a 2-stage process. Initially right-sided heart failure occurs secondary to severe pulmonary vasoconstriction, leading to volume and pressure overload with relatively preserved left heart function. This step is followed by left heart failure in the second stage, possibly due to myocardial ischemia or a direct myocardial depressant effect of amniotic fluid or other mediators. In support of this 2-stage theory, cardiopulmonary bypass (CPB) has been used successfully in at least 1 case of early AFE to off-load the right heart and prevent the progression to left-sided heart failure.[35] This patient was weaned from CPB after 83 minutes, extubated in the intensive care unit on postpartum day (PPD) 1, and was discharged from the hospital on PPD 7, with only some peripartum memory loss and exacerbation of her previously existing carpal tunnel syndrome. If readily available, TTE is a valuable tool in the diagnosis of AFE, which may help prevent the progression to full cardiovascular collapse and maternal death.

DIFFERENTIAL DIAGNOSIS

The differential diagnosis of AFE is extensive and includes thromboembolism or air embolism, transfusion reaction, hemorrhage, anaphylaxis, placental abruption, uterine rupture, cardiomyopathy, eclampsia, acute myocardial infarction, septic shock, and high spinal anesthesia (**Box 3**). With mortality rates up to 90% and neurologic sequelae in 85% of survivors,[5] better ways to define, diagnose, and treat AFE are continuously under study to find a way to prevent future maternal deaths.

TREATMENT

Most of the treatment efforts in AFE management are directed toward cardiovascular support, including maintaining adequate blood pressure, cardiac output, oxygenation, and tissue perfusion. Ideally this treatment should take place in an intensive care unit with appropriate monitoring, including cardiac telemetry to detect arrhythmias, continuous respiratory monitoring via pulse oximetry or end-tidal CO_2 if the patient is intubated, and continuous blood pressure monitoring with an arterial line. A pulmonary artery catheter may also be helpful for monitoring and trending cardiac output, central venous pressure, systemic vascular resistance, pulmonary artery pressure, and pulmonary capillary wedge pressure.[36,37] Use of vasopressors such as dopamine or norepinephrine may be required to maintain adequate perfusion, and the addition of

---

Box 3
Differential diagnosis for amniotic fluid embolism

Thromboembolism

Air embolism

Transfusion reaction

Hemorrhage

Anaphylaxis

Placental abruption

Uterine rupture

Cardiomyopathy

Myocardial infarction

Eclampsia

Septic shock

High spinal anesthesia

inotropes such as dobutamine and milrinone may help because of their β-adrenergic agonism, improvement of myocardial contractility, and α-adrenergic vasoconstrictor effects. Electrolyte and glucose imbalances also occur, and should be managed appropriately. Intravenous steroid administration may also be necessary following an AFE, secondary to disruption of the hypothalamic-pituitary axis as a result of massive hemorrhage secondary to DIC, causing a pan-hypopituitary state (Sheehan syndrome).[5]

Any coagulopathy must also be corrected to prevent obstetric hemorrhage. As hemorrhage occurs colloid replacement, especially packed red blood cells to help maintain oxygen delivery to the tissues, may be necessary and is considered first-line treatment for correcting the coagulopathy associated with AFE. Fibrinogen replacement has been shown to be especially important in massive transfusion for obstetric hemorrhage.[38] Cryoprecipitate, which contains fibronectin, could help facilitate removal of amniotic fluid debris from the circulation via monocyte and macrophage activity.[39,40]

Other treatment methods have been suggested but have yet to be thoroughly investigated. Administration of inhaled nitric oxide[41] or aerosolized prostacyclin for the treatment of severe hypoxemia,[42] aprotinin,[43,44] the serine protease inhibitor FOY-305 to treat DIC,[45] high-dose corticosteroids, hemodiafiltration to eliminate amniotic fluid from the blood,[46] exchange transfusion,[47] extracorporeal membrane oxygenation,[48] cardiopulmonary bypass,[49] uterine artery embolization,[50,51] pulmonary artery thrombectomy[52] and thrombolysis with tissue-plasminogen activator,[53] and intra-aortic balloon counterpulsation[48] all have been used for AFE.

Recently, the use of intralipid for the treatment of AFE has been suggested.[54] Since it was first investigated in 1998 in the resuscitation of rats suffering from cardiovascular collapse caused by bupivacaine toxicity, intralipid has been shown to be effective not only in local anesthetic toxicity but also for several other drug toxicities including calcium-channel blockers, antipsychotics, and tricyclic antidepressants. The mechanism in each case is thought to be the creation of a "lipid sink" that binds lipophilic drugs and transports them away from the site of action of the toxicity. Intralipid has also been shown to not only help prevent pulmonary hypertension and resultant right heart failure by a variety of mechanisms, but also to treat it when it is preexisting. As AFE is likely a result of circulating mediators causing pulmonary vasoconstriction leading to cardiovascular collapse, the hypothesis that intralipid, which has been shown to prevent the cascade that leads to pulmonary hypertension and right heart failure, may be used in the treatment of AFE is novel, and requires further investigation in animal models.

Another new, but somewhat controversial treatment of AFE is the use of recombinant factor VIIa,[55] specifically to help stop hemorrhage secondary to DIC. Factor VIIa activates the extrinsic coagulation pathway by combining with tissue factor, which is usually found in very low concentrations in the blood. When there is damage to a blood vessel, tissue factor is released and is exposed to circulating factor VIIa, which starts the cascade, resulting in fibrin deposition. Recombinant factor VIIa has been used successfully to treat postpartum hemorrhage in patients with abnormal placentation, uterine atony, and uterine rupture. However, in these conditions there are minimally increased levels of circulating tissue factor in comparison with AFE, where there are markedly higher circulating levels as a result of the consumptive nature of the DIC. If recombinant factor VIIa were used in AFE, inappropriate fibrin deposition theoretically would occur throughout the body, including the brain, kidneys, and heart. The package insert for recombinant factor VIIa specifically mentions an increased risk of developing thrombotic events if administered to patients with DIC (by definition present in patients with AFE).

A 2011 literature review by Leighton and colleagues[55] compared outcomes between patients with AFE who had received recombinant factor VIIa as part of their treatment in a comparison with those who did not. Despite the patient demographics and other resuscitation techniques used being similar, the patients who received factor VIIa had significantly worse outcomes (major organ thrombosis and death) than those who did not. Given that this is a retrospective analysis so that no causal relationship may be established, it does pose the question of whether it is appropriate to administer this prothrombotic agent to a patient with DIC secondary to AFE. While recognizing the limitations of a literature review and the possibility of selection bias, the investigators suggest that perhaps recombinant factor VIIa should be reserved only for patients in whom massive balanced blood component transfusion, including packed red blood cells, fresh frozen plasma, platelets, cryoprecipitate, and even fibrinogen, does not stop the hemorrhage.

OUTCOMES

Maternal outcome following AFE is not promising. The majority of cases result in death for the mother. Maternal mortality ranges from 44% to 61%, depending on the severity of the disease.[56] Mortality ratios range from 0.4 per 100,000 live births in the Netherlands to 1.3 per 100,000 live births in the United States.[57] Comparing the incidence of death from AFE with that from pulmonary embolism, the ratio of survivors to death is 2.3:1 versus 19:1. Kayem and colleagues[58] investigated risk factors for death from AFE. In their analysis they compared 476 women who survived and 100 women who died. Maternal death was associated with maternal age older than 35 years (odds ratio [OR] 2.36), black ethnicity (OR 2.38), and obesity as defined by a body mass index greater than 30 kg/m^2 (OR 2.73). If the risk factors are combined, the OR associated with death for all 3 risk factors is 4.4 (95% confidence interval 1.76–11.0). Another study that also examined fatal and nonfatal cases of AFE included 65 cases of fatal AFE and 70 nonfatal ones. Risk factors for fatal AFE were multiparity, noncesarean section at full-term, and the presence of 1 of the following: cardiac arrest, dyspnea, or loss of consciousness. Another interesting finding from the study was that levels of Sialyl Tn were higher in the serum of patients with fatal AFE. This result is not surprising, as Sialyl Tn is found in meconium. The higher serum level suggests that that the amount of meconium in the maternal serum was higher.[59] Fatality is associated with a greater influx of meconium into the maternal serum. The problem with determining the outcome lies with the diagnosis. To determine the outcome, the patient must be diagnosed with AFE. Given the difficulty in achieving the diagnosis, the ability to determine outcomes is hindered.

There is limited information on maternal outcome if the mother survives. If the patient survives the event, the outcome remains poor. Approximately 10% will be neurologically intact.[56] In the United Kingdom, 6% of patients with AFE who survived had cerebral injury, whereas in Australia 20% experienced stroke. Woman with AFE have a high incidence of blood transfusion, plasma transfusion, and hysterectomy. There is no difference in the incidence of these occurrences between nonfatal and fatal AFE. Of those who do survive AFE, approximately 50% will be discharged within 4 to 7 days while the remainder require a hospital stay of longer than 8 days.

There is also a paucity of information on infant outcomes in mothers who experience AFE. The largest reported series concerns 54 infants born to 120 mothers who met the criteria of AFE. Of this group, approximately 25% died in utero or after delivery. The surviving infants suffered from bacterial sepsis, seizures, and jaundice. More than 50% of the surviving infants required a hospital stay longer than 7 days.[60]

SUMMARY

AFE is an rare and lethal clinical syndrome, and is included in the differential diagnosis of any patient in the peripartum period who experiences sudden cardiovascular collapse, signs or symptoms of hypoxia, or hemorrhage. Despite an improved understanding of the etiology and pathophysiology of AFE, it remains one of the major causes of maternal morbidity and mortality in the United States. Advancements in diagnosis have led to several promising techniques, such as TEE and measurement of IGFBP1, which may help bring AFE from a diagnosis of exclusion to one that is clearly defined and testable in a rapid and reliable manner. Treatment remains supportive in nature by maintaining adequate tissue perfusion pressures and oxygenation, but may eventually include innovative modalities currently being investigated to help prevent or control the cardiopulmonary and hematologic derangements seen in AFE.

REFERENCES

1. Steiner PE, Lushbaugh CC. Landmark article, October 1941: maternal pulmonary embolism by amniotic fluid as a result of obstetric shock and unexpected deaths in obstetrics. JAMA 1986;255:2187–203.
2. Clark SL, Pavlova Z, Greenspoon J, et al. Squamous cells in the maternal pulmonary circulation. Am J Obstet Gynecol 1986;154(1):104–6.
3. Conde-Agudelo A, Romero R. Amniotic fluid embolism: an evidence-based review. Am J Obstet Gynecol 2009;201:445.e1–13.
4. Courtney LD. Amniotic fluid embolism. BMJ 1970;1:545.
5. Worly B, Butler JR. Amniotic fluid embolism. Postgrad Obstet Gynecol 2012; 32(12):1–5.
6. Abenhaim HA, Azoulay L, Kramer MS, et al. Incidence and risk factors of amniotic fluid embolisms: a population-based study on 3 million births in the United States. Am J Obstet Gynecol 2008;199:49.e1–8.
7. Knight M, UKOSS. Amniotic fluid embolism: active surveillance versus retrospective database review. Am J Obstet Gynecol 2008;199:e9.
8. Gilbert WM, Danielsen B. Amniotic fluid embolism: decreased mortality in a population- based study. Obstet Gynecol 1999;93:973–7.
9. Kramer MS, Rouleau J, Baskett TF, et al, Maternal Health Study Group of the Canadian Perinatal Surveillance System. Amniotic- fluid embolism and medical induction of labour: a retrospective, population-based cohort study. Lancet 2006;368:1444–8.
10. Samuelsson E, Hellgren M, Högberg U. Pregnancy-related deaths due to pulmonary embolism in Sweden. Acta Obstet Gynecol Scand 2007;86:435–43.
11. Pallasmaa N, Ekblad U, Gissler M. Severe maternal morbidity and the mode of delivery. Acta Obstet Gynecol Scand 2008;87:662–8.
12. Hammerschmidt DE, Ogburn PL, Williams JE. Amniotic fluid activates complement. A role in amniotic fluid embolism syndrome? J Lab Clin Med 1984;104:901–7.
13. Benson MD. Nonfatal amniotic fluid embolism. Three possible cases and a new clinical definition. Arch Fam Med 1993;2:989–94.
14. Benson MD. A hypothesis regarding complement activation and amniotic fluid embolism. Med Hypotheses 2007;68:1019–25.
15. Benson MD, Kobayashi H, Silver RK, et al. Immunologic studies in presumed amniotic fluid embolism. Obstet Gynecol 2001;97:510–4.
16. Courtney LD, Allington M. Effect of amniotic fluid on blood coagulation. Br J Haematol 1972;22:353–5.

17. Østerud B, Bjørklid E. The tissue factor pathway in disseminated intravascular coagulation. Semin Thromb Hemost 2001;27:605–17.
18. Lockwood CJ, Bach R, Guha A, et al. Amniotic fluid contains tissue factor, a potent initiator of coagulation. Am J Obstet Gynecol 1991;165:1335–41.
19. Harnett MJ, Hepner DL, Datta S, et al. Effect of amniotic fluid on coagulation and platelet function in pregnancy: an evaluation using thromboelastography. Anaesthesia 2005;60:1068–72.
20. Liu EH, Shailaja S, Koh SC, et al. An assessment of the effects on coagulation of midtrimester and final trimester amniotic fluid on whole blood by thrombelastograph analysis. Anesth Analg 2000;90:333–6.
21. Clark SL, Hankins GD, Dudley DA, et al. Amniotic fluid embolism: analysis of the national registry. Am J Obstet Gynecol 1995;172:1158–69.
22. Lewis G. The confidential enquiry into maternal and child health (CEMACH). Saving mothers' lives: reviewing maternal deaths to make motherhood safer— 2002-2005. The seventh report on confidential enquiries into maternal deaths in the United Kingdom. London: CEMACH; 2007.
23. Roberts CL, Algert CS, Knight M, et al. Amniotic fluid embolism in an Australian population-based cohort. BJOG 2010;117:1417–21.
24. Sinicina I, Pankratz H, Bise K, et al. Forensic aspects of post-mortem histological detection of amniotic fluid embolism. Int J Legal med 2010;124: 55–62.
25. Kuhlman K, Hidvegi D, Tamura RK, et al. Is amniotic fluid material in the central circulation of peripartum patients pathologic? Am J Perinatol 1985;2:295–9.
26. Marcus BJ, Collins KA, Harley RA. Ancillary studies in amniotic fluid embolism: a case report and review of the literature. Am J Forensic Med Pathol 2005;26: 92–5.
27. Kanayama N, Yamazaki T, Naruse H, et al. Determining zinc coproporphyrin in maternal plasma—a new method for diagnosis amniotic fluid embolism. Clin Chem 1992;38:526–9.
28. Legrand M, Rossignol M, Dreux S, et al. Diagnostic accuracy of insulin-like growth factor binding protein-1 for amniotic fluid embolism. Crit Care Med 2012;40:2059–63.
29. Shechtman M, Ziser A, Markovits R, et al. Amniotic fluid embolism: early findings of transesophageal echocardiography. Anesth Analg 1999;89:1456–8.
30. Gregory MG, Clayton EM Jr. Amniotic fluid embolism. Obstet Gynecol 1973;42: 236–44.
31. Grossman W, Braunwald E. Pulmonary hypertension. In: Braunwald E, editor. Heart disease. 2nd edition. Philadelphia: WB Saunders; 1984. p. 823–48.
32. Clark SL, Montz FJ, Phelan JP. Hemodynamic alterations associated with amniotic fluid embolism: a reappraisal. Am J Obstet Gynecol 1985;151:617–21.
33. Clark SL, Cotton DB, Gonik B, et al. Central hemodynamic alterations in amniotic fluid embolism. Am J Obstet Gynecol 1988;158:1124–6.
34. James CF, Feinglass NG, Menke DM, et al. Massive amniotic fluid embolism: diagnosis aided by emergency transesophageal echocardiography. Int J Obstet Anesth 2004;13:279–83.
35. Stanten RD, Iverson LI, Daugharty TM, et al. Amniotic fluid embolism causing catastrophic pulmonary vasoconstriction: diagnosis by transesophageal echocardiogram and treatment by cardiopulmonary bypass. Obstet Gynecol 2003; 102:496–8.
36. Moore J, Baldisser MR. Amniotic fluid embolism. Crit Care Med 2005;33: S279–85.

37. O'Shea A, Eappen S. Amniotic fluid embolism. Int Anesthesiol Clin 2007;45: 17–28.
38. de Lloyd L, Bovington R, Kaye A, et al. Standard haemostatic tests following major obstetric hemorrhage. Int J Obstet Anesth 2011;20(2):135–41.
39. Bastien JL, Graves JR, Bailey S. Atypical presentation of amniotic fluid embolism. Anesth Analg 1998;87:124–6.
40. Rodgers GP, Heymach GJ 3rd. Cryoprecipitate therapy in amniotic fluid embolization. Am J Med 1984;76:916–20.
41. McDonnell NJ, Chan BO, Frengley RW. Rapid reversal of critical haemodynamic compromise with nitric oxide in a parturient with amniotic fluid embolism. Int J Obstet Anesth 2007;16:269–73.
42. Van Heerden PV, Webb SA, Hee G, et al. Inhaled aerosolized prostacyclin as a selective pulmonary vasodilator for the treatment of severe hypoxaemia. Anaesth Intensive Care 1996;24:87–90.
43. Oney T, Schander K, Müller N, et al. Amniotic fluid embolism with coagulation disorder—a case report. Geburtshilfe Frauenheilkd 1982;42:25–8 [in German].
44. Stroup J, Haraway D, Beal JM. Aprotinin in the management of coagulopathy associated with amniotic fluid embolus. Pharmacotherapy 2006;26:689–93.
45. Taenaka N, Shimada Y, Kawai M, et al. Survival from DIC following amniotic fluid embolism. Successful treatment with a serine proteinase inhibitor; FOY. Anaesthesia 1981;36:389–93.
46. Kaneko Y, Ogihara T, Tajima H, et al. Continuous hemodiafiltration for disseminated intravascular coagulation and shock due to amniotic fluid embolism: report of a dramatic response. Intern Med 2001;40:945–7.
47. Dodgson J, Martin J, Boswell J, et al. Probable amniotic fluid embolism precipitated by amniocentesis and treated by exchange transfusion. Br Med J (Clin Res Ed) 1987;294:1322–3.
48. Hsieh YY, Chang CC, Li PC, et al. Successful application of extracorporeal membrane oxygenation and intra-aortic balloon counterpulsation as lifesaving therapy for a patient with amniotic fluid embolism. Am J Obstet Gynecol 2000;183:496–7.
49. Rufforny-Doudenko I, Sipp C, Shehata BM. Pathologic quiz case. A 30-year-old woman with severe disseminated intravascular coagulation during delivery. Arch Pathol Lab Med 2002;126:869–70.
50. Dorne R, Pommier C, Emery JC, et al. Amniotic fluid embolism: successful evolution course after uterine arteries embolization. Ann Fr Anesth Reanim 2002;21: 431–5 [in French].
51. Goldszmidt E, Davies S. Two cases of hemorrhage secondary to amniotic fluid embolus managed with uterine artery embolization. Can J Anaesth 2003;50: 917–21.
52. Esposito RA, Grossi EA, Coppa G, et al. Successful treatment of postpartum shock caused by amniotic fluid embolism with cardiopulmonary bypass and pulmonary artery thromboembolectomy. Am J Obstet Gynecol 1990;163:572–4.
53. Hosokawa S, Hiasa Y, Ogata T, et al. A survival case of amniotic fluid embolism treated by percutaneous cardiopulmonary support and thrombolysis with tissue-plasminogen activator. Nippon Naika Gakkai Zasshi 2001;90:2074–6 [in Japanese].
54. Eldor J, Kotlovker V. Intralipid for amniotic fluid embolism (AFE)? Open J Anesthesiol 2012;2.
55. Leighton BL, Wall MH, Lockhart EM, et al. Use of recombinant factor VIIa in patients with amniotic fluid embolism: a systematic review of case reports. Anesthesiology 2011;115(6):1201–8.

56. Clark SL. Amniotic fluid embolism. Clin Obstet Gynecol 2010;53:322–8.
57. Knight M, Berg C, Brocklehurst P, et al. Amniotic fluid embolism incidence, risk factors and outcomes: a review and recommendations. BMC Pregnancy Childbirth 2012;12:7–11.
58. Kayem G, Kurinczuk J, Lewis G, et al. Risk factors for progression from severe maternal morbidity to death: A national cohort study. PloS One 2011;6:e29077.
59. Oi H, Naruse K, Noguchi T, et al. Fatal factors of clinical manifestations and laboratory testing in patients with amniotic fluid embolism. Gynecol Obstet 2010; 70:138–44.
60. Kramer MS, Rouleau J, Liu S, et al. Amniotic fluid embolism: incidence, risk factors, and impact on perinatal outcome. BJOG 2012;119:874–9.

Inhaled Nitrous Oxide for Labor Analgesia

Sarah A. Starr, MD*, Curtis L. Baysinger, MD

KEYWORDS

- Nitrous oxide for labor • Labor analgesia • Entonox • Labor pain
- Inhalational analgesia • Systemic labor analgesia

KEY POINTS

- Nitrous oxide for labor is commonly used worldwide, with good safety for mother and infant.
- Inhaled nitrous oxide provides mild to moderate pain relief and anxiolysis for women in labor.
- The use of nitrous oxide as a sole agent at concentrations less than 50% is considered minimal sedation and does not require the continuous presence of an anesthesia provider.
- Maternal side effects occur frequently but are mild.
- Clinical success is highly dependent on adequate patient instruction.

INTRODUCTION

Inhaled nitrous oxide is the most commonly used labor analgesic in many countries. It is used for greater than 50% of births in Finland, Norway, England, Australia, and New Zealand; 70% of births in Sweden; and 60% of births in the United Kingdom.[1–3] Despite its established role in relief of labor pain in other countries, use of nitrous oxide for labor has been uncommon in the United States. Barriers to use in the United States include a lack of suitable equipment and provider unfamiliarity with the technique. A major obstacle to US use of nitrous oxide was recently lifted when Porter Instruments, a division of Parker-Hannifin (Hatfield, PA, USA) , began sales and shipping of a new Nitronox™ machine in 2013.[4] This product is being marketed to hospitals, medical centers, and birth facilities for use in labor (**Fig. 1**).

Funding Sources: None.

Conflicts of Interest: None.

Division of Obstetric Anesthesia, Department of Anesthesiology, Vanderbilt University Medical Center, 4202 VUH, Nashville, TN 37232, USA

* Corresponding author.

E-mail address: sarah.a.starr@vanderbilt.edu

Anesthesiology Clin 31 (2013) 623–634

http://dx.doi.org/10.1016/j.anclin.2013.04.001

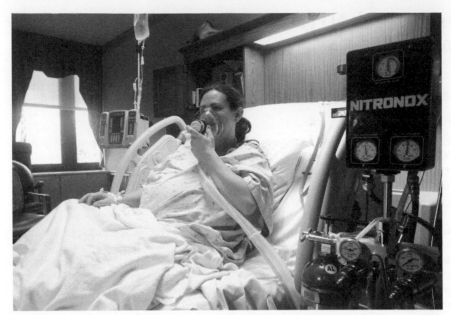

Fig. 1. Patient being administered nitrous oxide during labor.

The infrequent use of nitrous oxide for labor in the United States makes the development of standards difficult. In many countries, it is administered by midwives without anesthesia oversight.[5] Recent efforts to expand the use of nitrous oxide in the United States have emerged primarily from advocacy within the midwifery profession.[6] In the United States, it is administered by anesthesiologists in at least 3 academic settings and by either anesthesiologists or midwives in at least 1 other (Judith Bishop, personal communication, 2011).

Nitrous oxide is a tasteless and odorless gas at standard atmospheric pressure. It is a weak anesthetic with a minimum alveolar concentration (MAC) of 111%; it is frequently used in conjunction with other agents as part of a multiagent anesthetic technique.[4] Nitrous oxide is offered by up to 50% of US dentists for sedation, where it is inhaled continuously via a nasal mask at concentrations ranging from 30% to 70%.[7] In dentistry, it is typically used without pulse oximetry or other hemodynamic monitoring.[7]

Nitrous oxide is administered through the lungs by inhalation, and metabolism is negligible, with little accumulation in fat and other tissues. Onset and duration are both dose dependent, and excretion occurs via the pulmonary system as the agent is exhaled. The mechanism of action is complex and not well understood. Analgesia may result from central nervous system potassium channel inhibition[8] as well as release of endogenous opioids.[9] This process does not seem to involve μ receptor stimulation,[10] but may involve κ receptor activation.[11] Anxiolysis is mediated by γ-aminobutyric acid receptors, and N-methyl-D-aspartate (NMDA) inhibition is likely the mechanism for the weak dissociative effect of nitrous oxide.[8,12,13]

Nitrous oxide is self-administered and delivered through a face mask or mouthpiece. It is mixed with oxygen in a 50:50 ratio and is typically breathed intermittently, timed to uterine contractions. A rapid onset and offset are caused by its low solubility in blood; this rapid onset allows the patient to titrate the dose to the level of perceived pain. When discontinued, the effects of nitrous oxide disappear within a few minutes. Nitrous oxide at concentrations up to 50% is considered minimal sedation/analgesia when used as a sole agent and therefore does not require continuous monitoring by anesthesia personnel during its administration.[14] With minimal sedation, laryngeal reflexes are intact, and the patient should not have an increased risk of aspiration or respiratory depression. Fetal heart tones are unaffected, as is maternal oxygenation.[2]

HISTORY OF NITROUS OXIDE USE FOR LABOR

The invention of nitrous oxide is generally attributed to Joseph Priestly, who first synthesized this compound in 1772.[15] Experimentation with nitrous oxide in the early part of the eighteenth century was focused on its potential to cure disease. It did not do so, but was found to be a popular social intoxicant by Humphry Davy, whose demonstrations at the Institute for Pneumatic Medicine introduced this drug to eighteenth-century authors and dignitaries. Davy wrote of nitrous oxide's potential to relieve pain of surgery in his book published in 1800, but was not known to have advocated the gas for anesthetic use.[16] The use of nitrous oxide as an anesthetic was first suggested by dentist Horace Wells after he learned of the agent from traveling showman Gardner Quincy Colton.[17] However, Wells's formal demonstration of nitrous oxide for surgery in 1845 was a disappointment. A year later, the successful demonstration of anesthesia (with ether) by Wells's colleague William Morton took place at Massachusetts General Hospital; this monumental event is widely considered to mark the birth of anesthesia. The use of nitrous oxide as a sole anesthetic was largely abandoned, but use in dentistry (an indication for which it was arguably better suited) continued to increase and was popularized by Gardner Quincy Colton, who had first introduced Horace Wells to nitrous oxide.[17]

The first use of nitrous oxide for obstetrics is credited to Russian physician Stanislov Klikovich, who developed a machine that delivered 80% nitrous oxide with 20% oxygen.[18] Klikovich published the first study of nitrous oxide in laboring women in 1881, establishing its safety and effectiveness. However, widespread use of this agent in obstetrics did not follow, because the cost and cumbersome nature of equipment needed to deliver the nitrous oxide in combination with oxygen were prohibitive.

In the early twentieth century, several prototypical devices for self-administration were developed; the most widely used was the Minnitt apparatus introduced in 1933.[19] Delivering 50% nitrous oxide mixed with air, it was advocated as a safe method of pain relief for patients attended by midwives without the oversight of a physician. In 1961, the introduction of Entonox provided an additional measure of safety by combining nitrous oxide with oxygen rather than air in a premixed tank; machines delivering nitrous oxide with air were subsequently retired from service. Entonox continues to be used widely for nitrous oxide analgesia.[19,20]

EFFICACY OF INHALED NITROUS OXIDE FOR LABOR ANALGESIA

Studies of efficacy are limited and most are of poor quality. Most have compared nitrous oxide with other volatile agents or with itself at varying concentrations; placebo studies are few.[21,22] Carstoniu and colleagues[23] reported no significant difference in pain scores for 26 women breathing 50% nitrous oxide versus compressed air in a crossover trial. A limitation to the study was the lack of patient teaching to instruct participants to time breathing to contractions. A subsequent trial by Talebi and colleagues[24] using patient teaching reported a significant reduction in visual analogue scores of 20 mm when nitrous oxide was used compared with control (air). A recent Cochrane review of 890 studies of inhaled labor analgesia[25] reported that inhalational analgesia with volatile agents and nitrous oxide was clinically effective in reducing labor pain, although significant reductions in pain relief with nitrous oxide alone have not been proved. Despite a long history of clinical use, the evidence for efficacy remains largely unsubstantiated.[22] However, relief of pain alone may not be the most important contributor to benefit; observational studies of efficacy show that 40% to 50% of women who use it for analgesia for labor deliver without use of alternative methods of analgesia.[22]

SIDE EFFECTS OF INHALED NITROUS OXIDE USE

Inhaled nitrous oxide analgesia for labor has been used for several decades with good safety outcomes for both mother and child.[5] The respiratory depressant effect of nitrous oxide administration during labor has not been proven, although its use may increase the rate of physiologic maternal oxygen desaturation between labor contractions.[22,26–29] Meaningful conclusions are difficult because oxygen desaturation is known to occur during unmedicated labors.[22] One small study found rates of desaturation to be similar between women who received neuraxial analgesia and inhaled nitrous oxide.[30]

Use of nitrous oxide does not seem to appreciably affect rates of maternal nausea or vomiting during labor.[22,26] It can be useful to screen the patient for ongoing or recent nausea before starting nitrous oxide; nausea may respond to ondansetron or other antiemetics. Dizziness is common and has been reported at rates ranging from 6% to 23%.[2] Dizziness is typically well tolerated, but occasionally may be unacceptable, requiring discontinuation of use.

Adding systemic opioids to nitrous oxide analgesia may increase the incidence of maternal hypoxemia compared with that resulting from systemic opioids alone.[27,28] The clinical effect of mild maternal hypoxemia on the normal or mildly stressed fetus is unknown[26]; most studies have failed to show any significant effects on Apgar scores[22,31] or umbilical cord blood gases.[32]

Maternal drowsiness is reported to occur in 0% to 24% of laboring women,[22] and rates of maternal unconsciousness seem to increase in a dose-dependent fashion when nitrous oxide is administered with other sedating agents. Unconsciousness has been reported in 0% to 1% of patients when concentrations of 50% nitrous oxide are used with systemic opioids or inhaled volatile agents.[33–36] The few studies reporting unconsciousness outcomes when nitrous oxide is used as a sole agent have found a zero incidence of unconsciousness.[37,38]

The potential for nitrous oxide to accumulate in closed air spaces has been well documented,[39] and caution is advised before using it in women who have a previous history of pneumothorax, retinal surgery, or recent middle ear or sinus infection.[40–42] Caution in patients who have had previous retinal surgery is of particular concern, because severe visual loss has been shown in patients receiving nitrous oxide months after eye surgery involving gas injection.[42]

Concern over the neurotoxic effects of various anesthetic agents on the developing brain has been raised in response to studies showing neuroapoptosis in rodents[43] and primates exposed to various anesthetic agents at large doses.[44] NMDA antagonists including ketamine and nitrous oxide may be more likely to induce apoptotic changes when compared with other anesthetic agents.[45,46] The effects in human fetuses or in children later in life who were exposed to nitrous oxide or other anesthetic agents in utero is unknown.[47] Animal models that have elicited concern involved subjects exposed to concentrations and durations of agents higher than that typically used during general anesthesia.[48] The low concentrations and brief period to which a fetus would be exposed during labor (even a prolonged one) would be unlikely to result in measurable effect even if such effects were later shown to be real.

The importance of the reduction in methionine synthetase activity after nitrous oxide administration during general anesthesia has been debated for many years. Although reduced methionine synthetase activity has been reported in the placentas of healthy women who have received nitrous oxide analgesia, no harm or clinical effect has been reported as a result.[49] However, some special circumstances may warrant caution, because rare cases of subacute combined degeneration have been reported in severely B_{12}-deficient persons receiving nitrous oxide general anesthesia.[47] Individuals at increased risk for B_{12} deficiency include those with pernicious anemia, patients with a history of extensive bowel resection because of Crohn disease, and vegans who do not consume legumes.[47] In general, vegetarian patients are not considered at high risk for B_{12} deficiency, although any patient with a documented B_{12} deficiency should not use nitrous oxide for labor.

A COMPARISON OF NITROUS OXIDE ANALGESIA WITH OTHER METHODS OF LABOR ANALGESIA
Parenteral Opioids

Intravenous and intramuscular opioids are commonly used for labor pain.[21] The analgesic effect of nitrous oxide may be greater, because it is associated with moderate decreases in visual analogue pain scores of 20 mm.[22] Systemic opioids are associated with a maternal sedation. When given close to delivery, opioids can cause fetal respiratory depression and lowered Apgar scores,[21] and use in late labor is often restricted.[50] In contrast, nitrous oxide has been shown to have minimal fetal effects, and its use may be extended into the third stage of labor and for postdelivery surgical repair.[23]

Recent randomized trials have compared nitrous oxide with intravenous patient-controlled analgesia (PCA) with remifentanil. Remifentanil has a significantly faster onset of action and peak effect compared with other opioids, making it possible to administer intermittent bolus doses timed to contractions.[51,52] Volmanen and colleagues[53] reported a greater reduction in pain scores with remifentanil compared with nitrous oxide (mean reduction of 1.5 vs 0.5 points on a 0–10 visual analog scale) but also found increased maternal sedation scores with remifentanil compared with nitrous oxide (2.0 compared with 0.5 on a 0–3 Likert scale). Remifentanil may be an effective intermittent labor analgesic, but widespread use is limited by patient monitoring requirements and technical limitations of PCA delivery systems.[21]

Other Inhalational Anesthetics

Various inhaled volatile anesthetic gases have been used at low doses for intermittent labor analgesia and are effective and well tolerated.[25] Sevoflurane has been recently investigated and may be more effective than nitrous oxide for use in labor.[54,55] The use of volatile inhaled agents may be limited, because of concerns that uterine relaxation associated with volatile anesthetics may increase the risk for postdelivery bleeding.[56]

Epidural Analgesia

Epidural analgesia is the most common labor analgesic used in the United States (approximately 61% of vaginal deliveries in 2008).[57] Regional analgesia with local anesthetics provides the most effective relief of labor pain, with reductions of 50 mm on visual analogue pain scales noted in most studies.[58] Although no randomized controlled trials have compared nitrous oxide analgesia with epidural analgesia for labor, the reductions in pain score with regional techniques are associated with high levels of maternal satisfaction.[59]

However, an overall failure rate of 12% and need for catheter replacement in 6.8% of neuraxial catheters (multiple times in up to 1.5% of patients),[60] as well as uncommon risks, including spinal headache and transient nerve irritation, may be reasons why some women select an alternative technique.[22] Inhaled nitrous oxide has no effect on uterine contractility and is not expected to affect the incidence of cesarean section, or length of any stage of labor.[2] Similarly, epidural analgesia does not increase the rate of cesarean birth nor does it prolong the first stage of labor, although slight prolongation of the second stage of labor may occur.[61]

ALTERNATIVE METHODS OF LABOR ANALGESIA

Hydrotherapy, relaxation and visualization techniques, transcutaneous electrical nerve stimulation (TENS), acupuncture, and acupressure have been used for labor analgesia.[62] The analgesic efficacy of these modalities are not established and not likely to provide greater efficacy compared with nitrous oxide.[25,62,63] One nonrandomized study compared nitrous oxide with TENS, meperidine, promethazine, and epidural analgesia and reported superior pain relief associated with epidural analgesia; 90% of women reported partial relief with nerve stimulation or nitrous oxide, whereas 54% reported partial pain relief with meperidine/promazine.[22,64] There are no studies comparing nitrous oxide with pudendal block for the relief of pain during the second stage of labor. Paracervical block is not widely used for labor analgesia, because of the high incidence of fetal heart rate abnormalities that accompany the block, despite recent improvements in technique designed to improve its safety.[65]

CLINICAL USE

Nitrous oxide is indicated for the relief of pain of labor and delivery, and for repair of lacerations after birth. It may also be used for other peripartum procedures such as uterine eversion and repair of cervical lacerations. Procedures for the administration of inhaled nitrous oxide for labor should comply with department anesthesia sedation policies in each institution in which it is used. In the United States, these policies should follow Centers for Medicare and Medicaid Services guidelines for anesthesia care.[66] Health care facilities should develop written protocols for use and have pulse oximetry and gas scavenging systems available.[22]

The American Society of Anesthesiologists practice guidelines for sedation and analgesia categorize nitrous oxide administration alone in concentrations less than 50% as analgesia or minimal sedation.[14] Therefore, when self-administered by patients in labor, a 50% nitrous oxide in oxygen technique does not require continuous in-room monitoring by an anesthesia provider unless additional sedating agents are used. Patients who have received additional systemic opioids within 2 hours of nitrous oxide use should have continuous pulse oximetry monitoring.[5]

The success of nitrous oxide therapy depends on adequate patient instruction and may require significant coaching. Providers who initiate nitrous oxide therapy should be fully trained to adequately explain the technique and should remain with the patient for several contraction cycles to observe the patient's ability to use it properly and assess the clinical effect. Adequate analgesia depends on the patient sensing the early onset of her contraction and taking 4 or 5 slow consecutive deep breaths, ideally 30 to 45 seconds before the peak of the uterine contraction is felt. Providers should emphasize the importance of sensing the beginning of contractions, taking near vital capacity breaths, and maintaining good mask seal. Patients should complete the series of breaths without removing the mask from their face, thereby limiting room air entrainment and ambient accumulation of nitrous oxide. Patients should hold their own mask rather than have a helper apply the mask for them.

EQUIPMENT USED IN ADMINISTERING NITROUS OXIDE FOR LABOR

In Great Britain and other countries, nitrous oxide equipment often consists of a single tank of nitrous oxide/oxygen connected to a demand valve and mask. In the United States, single tank systems are not used. One machine suitable for obstetric use is currently available in the United States. The Nitronox™ machine combines separate nitrous oxide and oxygen sources in a blender device and delivers a preset concentration of 50% nitrous oxide. This machine can use both wall and e-cylinder tank sources of nitrous oxide and oxygen. The use of tank oxygen requires frequent replacement, and wall oxygen is typically a better alternative when it is available. Tank nitrous oxide is largely liquid and provides a long duration of use, making the need for wall source nitrous oxide less important. A scavenger unit is integral to the machine and actively suctions exhaled gas for evacuation via a standard wall suction port. A demand valve located at the distal end of the circuit is connected to a disposable face mask or mouthpiece. The demand valve limits the high-pressure gas flow to occur only during active inhalation, allowing for deep breaths timed to contractions unique to use in labor. Because nitrous oxide is typically breathed intermittently, the demand valve also prevents leakage of nitrous oxide into the ambient environment when the patient is not using the device between contractions.

Pressurized nitrous oxide exists in a partially liquid state. The liquid portion of nitrous oxide does not exert pressure, and thus tank pressure remains steady at approximately 750 PSI until all liquid in the tank is depleted. At this point, tank pressure begins to decrease rapidly (and most of the tank volume has gone). The pressure gauge of nitrous oxide tanks should be monitored during use and the tank replaced when the gauge pressure reads 500 PSI. Frequent monitoring serves to minimize the risk of tank depletion during patient use.

ENVIRONMENTAL IMPLICATIONS OF NITROUS OXIDE USE

The amount of exhaled nitrous oxide released into the labor room environment should be minimized; amounts should be consistent with published Occupational Safety and Health Administration (OSHA) advisory guidelines regarding anesthetic gases in the work place.[67] When methods to scavenge exhaled gas are not used, health care workers may be exposed to nitrous oxide levels that exceed recommended standards.[26,45,46] However, establishing a measurable risk to health care providers is difficult, because potential long-term adverse effects of worker exposure to nitrous oxide remain unclear.[22,46,56]

Nitronox equipment uses a highly efficient scavenging system that uses wall suction to remove exhaled nitrous oxide. This system reduces environmental exposure lower than recommended levels where it has been tested (JT Bishop, personal communication, 2011) and is likely superior to the ventilation and limited scavenging techniques currently used in the United Kingdom.

OSHA recommends air sampling for anesthetic gases every 6 months to measure worker exposures and check effectiveness of control measures.[67] Personal nitrous oxide passive dosimeters are available but have not been validated by OSHA. Periodic sampling of nitrous oxide in labor wards is not specifically addressed.

NITROUS OXIDE AS A GREENHOUSE GAS

Nitrous oxide is a potent greenhouse gas, but medical emissions of nitrous oxide comprise only a small proportion of the total sources of greenhouse gases.[1] Thus, the value of scavenging nitrous oxide in reducing overall greenhouse gas emission is limited. Swedish manufacturers of nitrous oxide machinery have been proactive in the development of nitrous oxide delivery systems equipped with destruction units capable of reclaiming and destroying nitrous oxide to minimize its release into the environment. These units have been remarkably effective in limiting nitrous oxide emissions in Sweden. Ek and Tjus[1] reported that 33,386 kg of medical N_2O emissions were released in Sweden in 2002 before introduction of these units and that by 2010 that figure had been reduced to 15,959 kg. The introduction of destruction units into other countries may be slow, because of the high cost and large size of the equipment required for this purpose.

SUMMARY

Inhaled nitrous oxide has a long history of safe use for labor analgesia. Although its analgesic efficacy in laboring women has not been clearly established and it provides less effective pain relief when compared with neuraxial analgesia; it offers a good alternative to women who desire nonregional pain relief for labor and birth. Where epidurals are readily available, slightly more than one-half of patients using nitrous oxide deliver without conversion to regional analgesia.[22] Adverse effects are minimal and in general limited to mild side effects. Although safe administration requires the establishment of protocols, personnel training, and environmental monitoring practices, hemodynamic monitoring and continuous attendance by an anesthesia provider during administration are not required. Areas of further investigation in its use include techniques to improve the timing of administration to better coincide with the pain of uterine contraction; safety of administration by nonanesthesia personnel; the efficacy of additional coadministered methods to improve its analgesia; and the development of methods to better measure the improvement of maternal well-being during labor beyond pain relief.[22] Inhaled nitrous oxide provides a useful management tool that significantly improves analgesia and the birth experience for many women.

REFERENCES

1. Ek M, Tjus K. Destruction of medical N_2O in Sweden. In: Guoxiang L, editor. Greenhouse gasses–capturing, utilization and reduction. Shanghai (China): InTech; 2012. p. 185–98.
2. Likis FE, Andrews JA, Collins MR, et al. Nitrous oxide for the management of labor pain. Comparative effectiveness review no. 67. AHRQ publication no. 12-EHC071-EF. Rockville (MD): Agency for Healthcare Research and Quality; 2012. Available at:. http://www.effectivehealthcare.ahrq.gov/reports/final.cfm. Accessed March 21, 2013.
3. Fernando R, Jones T. Systemic analgesia: parenteral and inhalational agents. In: Chestnut DH, Polley LS, Wong C, editors. Obstetric anesthesia: principles and practice. 3rd edition. Philadelphia: Mosby Elsevier; 2009. p. 415–27.
4. Collins MR, Starr SA, Bishop JT, et al. Nitrous oxide for labor analgesia: expanding analgesic options for women in the United States. Rev Obstet Gynecol 2012; 5:e126–31.
5. Munro J. Understanding pharmacological pain relief. In: Royal College of Midwives, editors. Evidence based guidelines for midwifery-led care in labour.

2012. Available at: http://www.rcm.org.uk/college/policy-practice/evidence-based-guidelines. Accessed March 31, 2013.

6. Bishop JT. Administration of nitrous oxide in labor: expanding the options for women. J Midwifery Womens Health 2007;52:308–9.

7. Clark MS, Brunick AL. Signs and symptoms of N_2O/O_2 sedation. In: Dolan J, editor. Handbook of nitrous oxide and oxygen sedation. 3rd edition. St Louis (MO): Mosby Elsevier; 2008. p. 117–23.

8. Gruss M, Bushell TJ, Bright DP, et al. Two-pore-domain K^+ channels are a novel target for the anesthetic gases xenon, nitrous oxide, and cyclopropane. Mol Pharmacol 2004;65:443–52.

9. Duarte R, McNeill A, Drummond G, et al. Comparison of the sedative, cognitive, and analgesic effects of nitrous oxide, sevoflurane, and ethanol. Br J Anaesth 2008;100:203–10.

10. Koyama T, Mayahara T, Wakamatsu T, et al. Deletion of mu-opioid receptor in mice does not affect the minimum alveolar concentration of volatile anaesthetics and nitrous oxide-induced analgesia. Br J Anaesth 2009;103: 744–9.

11. Koyama T, Fukuda K. Involvement of the kappa-opioid receptor in nitrous oxide-induced analgesia in mice. J Anesth 2010;24:297–9.

12. Yamakura T, Harris RA. Effects of gaseous anesthetics nitrous oxide and xenon on ligand-gated ion channels. Comparison with isoflurane and ethanol. Anesthesiology 2000;93:1095–101.

13. Jevtović-Todorović V, Todorović SM, Mennerick S, et al. Nitrous oxide (laughing gas) is an NMDA antagonist, neuroprotectant and neurotoxin. Nat Med 1998;4: 383–4.

14. American Society of Anesthesiologists Task Force on Sedation and Analgesia by Non-Anesthesiologists. Practice guidelines for sedation and analgesia by non-anesthesiologists. Anesthesiology 2002;96:1004–17.

15. Frost EA. A history of nitrous oxide. In: Eger EI, editor. Nitrous oxide/N_2O. New York: Elsevier; 1985. p. 1–22.

16. Davy H. Conclusion. In: Researches, chemical and philosophical; chiefly concerning nitrous oxide, or dephlogosticated nitrous air, and its respiration. London: Biggs and Cottle for J Johnson; 1800. p. 548–9.

17. Cartwright FF. The English pioneers of anaesthesia (Beddoes, Davy, and Hickman). Baltimore (MD): Williams & Wilkins; 1953. p. 33.

18. Richards W, Parbrook GD, Wilson J. Stanislov Klikovich: pioneer of nitrous oxide and oxygen analgesia. Anaesthesia 1976;31:933–40.

19. O'Sullivan EP. Dr Robert James Minnitt 1889-1974: a pioneer of inhalational analgesia. J R Soc Med 1989;82:309–13.

20. Tunstall ME. Use of a fixed nitrous oxide and oxygen mixture from one cylinder. Lancet 1961;2:964.

21. Jones L, Othman M, Dowswell T, et al. Pain management for women in labour: an overview of systematic reviews. Cochrane Database Syst Rev 2012;(3):CD009234. http://dx.doi.org/10.1002/14651858.

22. Rosen MA. Nitrous oxide for relief of labor pain: a systematic review. Am J Obstet Gynecol 2002;186(Suppl):S110–26.

23. Carstoniu J, Levytam S, Norman P, et al. Nitrous oxide in early labor-safety and analgesic efficacy assessed by a double-blind, placebo-controlled study. Anesthesiology 1994;80:30–5.

24. Talebi H, Nourozi A, Jamilian M, et al. Entonox for labor pain: a randomized placebo controlled trial. Pak J Biol Sci 2009;12:1217–21.

25. Klomp T, van Poppel M, Jones L, et al. Inhaled analgesia for pain management in labour. Cochrane Database Syst Rev 2012;(9):CD009351. http://dx.doi.org/10.1002/14651858.

26. Yentis SM. The use of Entonox for labour pain should be abandoned. Proposer. Int J Obstet Anesth 2001;10:25–9.

27. Lucas DN, Siemaszko O, Yentis SM. Maternal hypoxaemia associated with the use of Entonox in labour. Int J Obstet Anesth 2000;9:270–2.

28. Deckardt R, Fembacher PM, Schneider KT, et al. Maternal arterial oxygen saturation during labor and delivery: pain-dependent alterations and effects on the newborn. Obstet Gynecol 1987;70:21–5.

29. Northwood D, Sapsford DJ, Jones JG, et al. Nitrous oxide sedation causes post-hyperventilation apnoea. Br J Anaesth 1991;67:7–12.

30. Arfeen A, Armstrong PJ, Whitfield A. The effects of Entonox and epidural analgesia on arterial oxygen saturation of women in labour. Anaesthesia 1994;49: 32–4.

31. Stefani S, Hughes S, Schnider S, et al. Neonatal neurobehavioral effects of inhalation analgesia for vaginal delivery. Anesthesiology 1982;56:351–5.

32. Griffin RP, Reynolds F. Maternal hypoxaemia during labour and delivery: the influence of analgesia and effect on neonatal outcome. Anaesthesia 1995;50: 151–6.

33. McAneny T, Doughty AG. Self-administered nitrous-oxide/oxygen analgesia in obstetrics. Anaesthesia 1963;18:488–97.

34. Ross JA, Tunstall ME, Campbell DM, et al. The use of 0.25% isoflurane premixed in 50% nitrous oxide and oxygen for pain relief in labour. Anaesthesia 1999;54: 1166–72.

35. Soyannwo OA. Self-administered Entonox (50% nitrous oxide in oxygen) in labour: report of the experience in Ibadan. Afr J Med Med Sci 1985;14: 95–8.

36. Jones PL, Rosen M, Mushin WW, et al. Methoxyflurane and nitrous oxide as obstetric analgesics. I. A comparison by continuous administration. Br Med J 1969;3(5665):255–9.

37. Arthurs GJ, Rosen M. Self-administered intermittent nitrous oxide analgesia for labour. Enhancement of effect with continuous nasal inhalation of 50 percent nitrous oxide (Entonox). Anaesthesia 1979;34:301–9.

38. Westling F, Milsom I, Zetterstrom H, et al. Effects of nitrous oxide/oxygen inhalation on the maternal circulation during vaginal delivery. Acta Anaesthesiol Scand 1992;36:175–81.

39. Munson ES. Transfer of nitrous oxide into body air cavities. Br J Anaesth 1974; 46:202–9.

40. Doyle WJ, Banks JM. Middle ear pressure change during controlled breathing with gas mixtures containing nitrous oxide. J Appl Phys 2003;94:199–204.

41. Eger EI, Saidman LJ. Hazards of nitrous oxide anesthesia in bowel obstruction and pneumothorax. Anesthesiology 1965;26:61–9.

42. Fu AD, McDonald HR, Eliott D, et al. Complications of general anesthesia using nitrous oxide in eyes with pre-existing gas bubbles. Retina 2002;22:569–74.

43. Creely CE, Olney JW. The young: neuroapoptosis induced by anesthetics and what to do about it. Anesth Analg 2010;110:442–8.

44. Bambrink AM, Evers AS, Avidan MS, et al. Isoflurane-induced neuroapoptosis in the neonatal rhesus macaque brain. Anesthesiology 2010;112:834–41.

45. Sanders RD, Weimann J, Maze M. Biologic effects of nitrous oxide. Anesthesiology 2008;109:707–22.

46. Mills GG, Singh D, Longan M, et al. Nitrous oxide exposure on the labour ward. Int J Obstet Anesth 1996;5:160–4.
47. Rosener M, Dichgans J. Severe combined degeneration of the spinal cord after nitrous oxide anaesthesia in a vegetarian. J Neurol Neurosurg Psychiatr 1996; 60:354.
48. Flood P. Fetal anesthesia and brain development. Anesthesiology 2011;114: 479–80.
49. Landon MJ, Creagh-Barry P, McArthur S, et al. Influence of vitamin B12 status on the inactivation of methionine synthase by nitrous oxide. Br J Anaesth 1992;69:81–6.
50. Halpern SH, Muir H, Breen TW, et al. A multicenter randomized controlled trial comparing patient-controlled epidural with intravenous analgesia for pain relief in labor. Anesth Analg 2004;99:1532–8.
51. Douma MR, Verwey RA, Kam-Endtz CE, et al. Obstetric analgesia: a comparison of patient-controlled meperidine, remifentanil, and fentanyl in labour. Br J Anaesth 2010;104:209–15.
52. Arnal D, Serrano ML, Corral EM, et al. Intravenous remifentanil for labor analgesia. Rev Esp Anestesiol Reanim 2009;56:222–31.
53. Volmanen P, Akural E, Raudaskoski T, et al. Comparison of remifentanil and nitrous oxide in labour analgesia. Acta Anaesthesiol Scand 2005;49:453–8.
54. Yeo ST, Holdcroft A, Yentis A, et al. Analgesia with sevoflurane during labour: determination of the optimum concentration. Br J Anaesth 2007;98: 105–9.
55. Yeo ST, Holdcroft A, Yentis SM, et al. Analgesia with sevoflurane during labour: ii. Sevoflurane compared with Entonox for labour analgesia. Br J Anaesth 2007; 98:110–5.
56. Fernando R, Jones T. Systemic analgesia: parenteral and inhalational agents. In: Chestnut DH, Polley LS, Tsen LC, et al, editors. Chestnut's obstetric anesthesia: principles and practice. 3rd edition. Philadelphia: Mosby Elsevier; 2009. p. 415–27.
57. Osterman MJ, Martin JA. Epidural and spinal anesthesia use during labor: 27-state reporting area. In: National vital statistics reports. vol. 59. 2008. p. 5. Available at: http://www.cdc.gov/nchs/data/nvsr/nvsr59/nvsr59_05.pdf. Accessed March 31, 2013.
58. Debiec J, Conell-Price J, Evansmith J, et al. Mathematical modeling of the pain and progress of the first stage of nulliparous labor. Anesthesiology 2009;111: 1093–110.
59. Wong CA. Epidural and spinal analgesia/anesthesia for labor and vaginal delivery. In: Chestnut DH, Polley LS, Tsen LC, et al, editors. Chestnut's obstetric anesthesia: principles and practice. Philadelphia: Mosby Elsevier; 2009. p. 429–92.
60. Pan PH, Bogard TD, Owen MD. Incidence and characteristics of failures in obstetric neuraxial analgesia and anesthesia: a retrospective analysis of 19,259 deliveries. Int J Obstet Anesth 2004;13:227–33.
61. Leighton BL, Halpern SH. The effects of epidural analgesia on labor, maternal, and neonatal outcomes. Am J Obstet Gynecol 2002;186:S69–77.
62. Smith CA, Levett KM, Collins CT, et al. Relaxation techniques for pain management in labour. Cochrane Database Syst Rev 2011;(12):CD009514. http://dx.doi.org/10.1002/14651858.
63. Cluett ER, Burns E. Immersion in water in labour and birth. Cochrane Database Syst Rev 2009;(2):CD000111. http://dx.doi.org/10.1002/14651858.

64. Harrison RF, Shore M, Woods T, et al. A comparative study of transcutaneous electrical nerve stimulation (TENS) entonox, pethidine + promazine, and lumbar epidural for pain relief in labor. Acta Obstet Gynecol Scand 1987;66:9–14.
65. Paech M. Newer techniques of labor analgesia. Anesthesiol Clin North America 2003;21:1–17.
66. Center for Medicaid and State Operations/Survey and Certification Group. Revised hospital anesthesia services interpretive guidelines–state operations manual (SOM) Appendix A. Baltimore (MD): Centers for Medicare and Medicaid Services; 2009.
67. Occupational safety and health guidelines for nitrous oxide. Occupational safety and health administration. 2010. Available at: http://www.osha.gov/SLTC/healthguidlines/nitrousoxide/recognition.html. Accessed March 31, 2013.

Index

Note: Page numbers of article titles are in **boldface** type.

A

Anesthesiology Clin 31 (2013) 635–643
http://dx.doi.org/10.1016/S1932-2275(13)00053-0
1932-2275/13/$ – see front matter © 2013 Elsevier Inc. All rights reserved.

Moving?

Make sure your subscription moves with you!

To notify us of your new address, find your **Clinics Account Number** (located on your mailing label above your name), and contact customer service at:

Email: journalscustomerservice-usa@elsevier.com

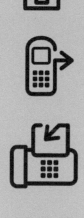

800-654-2452 (subscribers in the U.S. & Canada)
314-447-8871 (subscribers outside of the U.S. & Canada)

Fax number: 314-447-8029

Elsevier Health Sciences Division
Subscription Customer Service
3251 Riverport Lane
Maryland Heights, MO 63043

*To ensure uninterrupted delivery of your subscription, please notify us at least 4 weeks in advance of move.